Electronic Engineering for Neuromedicine

Online at: https://doi.org/10.1088/978-0-7503-3427-3

Electronic Engineering for Neuromedicine

Hussein Baher
Emeritus Professor of Electronic Engineering
Formerly with the Technological University of Dublin (TUD), Dublin, Ireland

IOP Publishing, Bristol, UK

ISBN 978-0-7503-3427-3 (ebook)
ISBN 978-0-7503-3425-9 (print)
ISBN 978-0-7503-3428-0 (myPrint)
ISBN 978-0-7503-3426-6 (mobi)

DOI 10.1088/978-0-7503-3427-3

Version: 20230101

IOP ebooks

British Library Cataloguing-in-Publication Data: A catalogue record for this book is available from the British Library.

Published by IOP Publishing, wholly owned by The Institute of Physics, London

IOP Publishing, No.2 The Distillery, Glassfields, Avon Street, Bristol, BS2 0GR, UK

US Office: IOP Publishing, Inc., 190 North Independence Mall West, Suite 601, Philadelphia, PA 19106, USA

Contents

Preface **viii**

Author biography **x**

1 An electronic perspective of the brain **1-1**

1.1 Introduction 1-1
1.2 The human brain 1-1
1.3 The cerebral cortex 1-3
1.4 The electronic nature of the brain 1-3
1.5 Modelling biological systems by electronic circuits 1-6
1.6 The logic of synthesis 1-8
1.7 Electric field theory 1-8
1.7.1 Capacitance 1-10
1.7.2 Electric current and current density 1-11
1.7.3 Displacement current 1-12
1.8 MOS transistors and microelectronic circuits 1-13
1.9 Conclusion 1-17
References 1-17

2 The brain as a signal processor **2-1**

2.1 Introduction 2-1
2.2 Signals and systems 2-1
2.3 Spectrum analysis 2-1
2.3.1 Correlation functions 2-5
2.3.2 Periodic signals 2-6
2.4 Modelling the brain 2-6
2.5 Accessing brain activity 2-8
2.5.1 Electroencephalography (EEG) 2-8
2.5.2 Implants 2-8
2.5.3 Electrocorticography (ECoG) 2-9
2.6 Brain–machine interface and cortex mapping 2-9
2.7 Conclusion 2-13
References 2-13

3 Neural signal processing **3-1**

3.1 Introduction 3-1
3.2 Neural signals 3-1

3.3	Filters and systems with frequency selectivity	3-2
3.4	Digitisation of analog signals	3-2
3.5	Digital filters	3-6
3.6	Stochastic (random) signals	3-6
	3.6.1 Probability distribution function	3-8
	3.6.2 Stationary processes	3-13
3.7	Power spectra of stochastic signals	3-13
	3.7.1 Cross-power spectrum	3-15
	3.7.2 White noise	3-15
3.8	Power spectrum estimation	3-15
3.9	Conclusion	3-17
	References	3-17
4	**Electronic psychiatry**	**4-1**
4.1	Introduction	4-1
4.2	Magnetic fields and electromagnetic field theory	4-1
	4.2.1 The Biot–Savart law (Laplace's rule)	4-2
	4.2.2 Ampere's circuital law	4-2
	4.2.3 Stokes' theorem	4-3
	4.2.4 The magnetic flux density	4-3
	4.2.5 Gauss' theorem	4-4
4.3	Vagus nerve stimulation (VNS)	4-6
4.4	Repetitive transcranial magnetic stimulation (rTMS)	4-8
4.5	Magnetic seizure therapy	4-9
4.6	Transcranial direct current stimulation (tDCS)	4-9
4.7	Deep brain stimulation (DBS)	4-10
4.8	Digital psychiatry	4-12
4.9	Conclusion	4-13
	References	4-13
5	**Neural engineering: merging neuroscience with engineering**	**5-1**
5.1	Introduction	5-1
5.2	Scanning and imaging techniques	5-1
5.3	Electromagnetic radiation and wave propagation	5-2
5.4	Magnetic resonance imaging (MRI)	5-2
	5.4.1 Resonance	5-2
	5.4.2 Dipoles	5-3

5.5	Blood supply ultrasound Doppler scans	5-6
5.6	Interaction of electric fields with neural tissue	5-7
5.7	Application in epilepsy	5-9
5.8	Electronics for paralysis	5-10
5.9	Artificial silicon retina	5-10
5.10	Cochlear implant	5-12
5.11	Electronic skin	5-13
5.12	Restoring the sense of touch	5-13
5.13	Robo surgeon	5-13
5.14	Electro-optic brain therapies	5-14
5.15	Neural prosthetics	5-14
5.16	Treatment of long Covid using electrical stimulation	5-15
5.17	Eavesdropping on the brain	5-15
5.18	Magnetoencephalography (MEG) using quantum sensors	5-16
5.19	Conclusion	5-16
	References	5-16

Preface

> *Science as it exists at present is partly agreeable, partly disagreeable. It is agreeable through the power it gives us of manipulating our environment, and to a small but important minority, it is agreeable because it affords intellectual satisfaction. It is disagreeable because, however we may seek to disguise the fact, it assumes a determinism which involves, theoretically, the power of predicting human actions; in this respect it seems to lessen human power.*
>
> —Bertrand Russell, 'Is Science Superstitious?' in *Sceptical Essays*

It is impossible to conceive of modern medicine without electronic engineering. Advances in electronics have revolutionised diagnostic tools and created mobile medicine, touch-sensitive prosthetics, remote surgery, artificial organs such as hearts and retinas, and bionic skins. Electronic engineers have also invented microsystems for drug implants and sensors for the early detection of disease. More often than not, what is perceived and described by the general public as a new advance in medicine is in fact a brilliant application of electronic engineering in the medical field.

Of particular strength is the connection between electronics and neuroscience. This is because it has been a two-way affair. In one direction, the brain has been modelled by electronic engineers as a collection of electronic circuit building blocks for the purposes of studying its function and diagnosis of its malfunctions. In the other direction the brain has repaid the electronics specialists by providing them with the ideas of artificial neural networks and artificial intelligence. This is now leading to efforts to understand and recreate human cognition which will probably give rise to significant advances in machine intelligence as well as having a great impact on neural medicine. It is certain that the cooperation between electronic engineers and neuroscientists will continue to intensify as more progress is made towards intelligent machines with increasing capabilities. *This book is concerned with the first aspect of this relationship, i.e. it deals with the areas of electronic engineering which are needed in neuromedicine and neuroscience.*

There are several ways in which electronic engineering feeds into neuromedicine:

1. The modelling and simulation of the brain in order to study its functions.
2. Providing access to the brain to extract information about its behaviour and for diagnostics.
3. Analysis of the signals and activities of the brain.
4. Influencing the function of the brain for therapeutic purposes either in an invasive or a non-invasive manner.
5. By a natural process one is led to some applications in psychiatry.

The areas of electronic engineering needed for understanding these applications are electronic circuits, spectral analysis, filtering of signals, electromagnetic fields, and wave propagation. The approach taken in this book is to integrate the electronics into the applications in neuromedicine in each chapter rather than give separate disjointed presentations of the two areas. For example, in a computer tomography machine (CT scan) or a magnetic resonance imaging (MRI) machine, all these areas are used in a complementary manner to arrive at the design of scanning and diagnostic tools that are only possible due to the advances in these areas of electronic engineering. Therefore, the full understanding of such methods is only possible with the understanding of these areas.

The book establishes in concrete terms the interplay between electronic engineering and neuroscience and provides some state-of-the-art ideas in electronic engineering which either have been established or have the potential and promise of becoming well established in medical practice. The book also illustrates by means of a number of typical representative examples, how engineering and neuroscience have merged to form the hybrid discipline of neural engineering.

The choice of material has followed two main principles. First, the selected application must be instructive; in other words, it must highlight ideas which have a general validity leading to the understanding of more than just the application at hand. Second, the significance of the application and its uses must be, in their broad outlines, accessible and interesting to the general public not just the specialist engineer or medical practitioner. After all, engineering and medicine share the distinction of being applied disciplines addressing themselves to the needs of humanity. It is hoped that the following goals will be achieved.

1. Medical students and practitioners will deepen their knowledge of electronic engineering, thus enhancing their understanding of the techniques lying behind the applications in neuromedicine.
2. Electronic engineering and physics students and graduates will gain knowledge of the application of their fields of study in neuromedicine.
3. The general readers will gain an appreciation of the interconnection between electronic engineering and neuromedicine and obtain a good overview of the applications in everyday life.

Finally, the friendliness and cooperation of my commissioning editor Ms Ashley Gasque in the production of the book are greatly appreciated.

H Baher
Vienna and Alexandria

Author biography

Hussein Baher

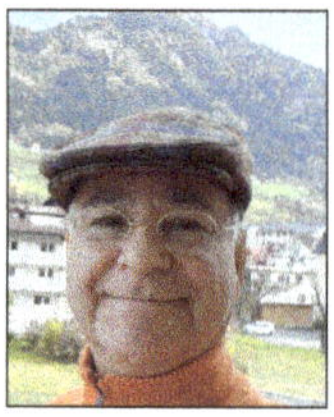

Professor Hussein Baher obtained his BSc in Engineering Electrophysics from Alexandria University, an MSc in Solid State Science from the American University in Cairo, and a PhD in Electronic Engineering from University College Dublin, Ireland. He specialised in the research areas of circuit theory, microwave engineering, microelectronics, and signal processing. He has occupied faculty positions at universities worldwide, including the Technological University of Dublin, University College Dublin, the first Professorship of Electronic Engineering at Dublin City University, Virginia Tech (USA), the Prestigious Analog Devices Chair of Microelectronics in Massachusetts (USA), as well as being a Visiting Professor at the Technical University of Vienna, Austria. In addition to numerous research papers in the areas of microelectronics and signal processing, he is the sole author of the books *Synthesis of Electrical Networks* (1984, Wiley), *Analog and Digital Signal Processing* (1990, Wiley), *Selective Linear Phase Switched-capacitor and Wave Digital Filters* (1993, Kluwer), *Microelectronic Switched-capacitor Filters, with ISICAP a Computer-aided Design Package* (1996, Wiley), *Analog and Digital Signal Processing* (2001, 2nd edn, Wiley), and *Signal Processing and Integrated Circuits* (2012, Wiley) which was translated into Chinese in 2015.

He is also interested in the application of electronic engineering in neuroscience and in Egyptology. On the latter subject, he has published the book *A Portrait of Egyptian Civilization* (2015, Lilith Publishing).

He is a Life Senior Member of the IEEE (USA) and a Fellow of the Electromagnetics Academy (Cambridge, MA, USA). He lives in Vienna and Alexandria, devoting most of his time to writing, travel, music, and Egyptology.

IOP Publishing

Electronic Engineering for Neuromedicine

Hussein Baher

Chapter 1

An electronic perspective of the brain

1.1 Introduction

This chapter begins by introducing the human brain to the general reader then proceeds to the electronic nature of the brain. The chapter introduces some basic concepts of electronic engineering needed for the study of the brain. These are important to explain the nomenclature used throughout the book and the principal ideas of electronic engineering together with those of neuroscience, thus establishing a common language. The idea of *modelling* biological systems by means of electronic circuits is highlighted in a general sense by considering a model of parts of the auditory system which has a heavy neurological content. Then, electronic engineering is discussed as a design-oriented scientific discipline which relies on the *synthesis* of components to create a functioning system according to given specifications to perform a certain task. For medical professionals who seek a deep understanding of the foundations of electrical and electronic engineering, the sections on electric field theory and microelectronic circuits should be useful.

1.2 The human brain

Figure 1.1 shows a simplified cross-sectional view of the human brain looking into the right hemisphere [1]. The brain consists of the cerebrum, the cerebellum, and the brain stem. The cerebrum is dominated by the two paired hemispheres responsible for personality, language, behaviour, intelligence and emotions. The cerebellum is responsible for balance, muscle tone and coordination. The brain stem leads to the spinal cord, which is the other part of the central nervous system (CNS). The cerebral cortex is folded forming convolutions or *gyri*. It has four lobes: frontal, parietal, temporal and occipital, as shown in figure 1.1. The following are brief explanations of the areas shown in figure 1.1:

doi:10.1088/978-0-7503-3427-3ch1

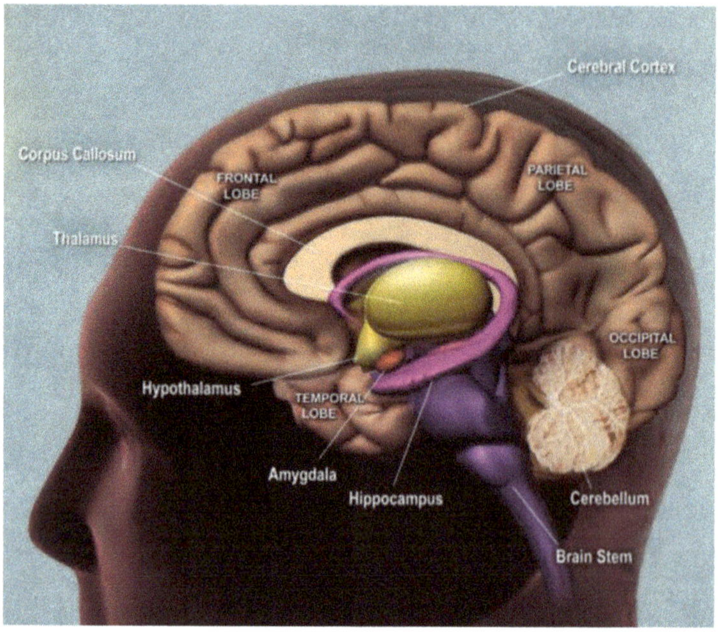

Figure 1.1. Simplified view into the right hemisphere of the human brain [1]. *Source*: National Institute on Aging https://commons.wikimedia.org/wiki/File:Side_View_of_the_Brain.png Public Domain.

a. The corpus callosum is a bundle of 200–300 million nerve fibres connecting the two brain hemispheres allowing communication between the two sides of the brain.
b. The frontal lobe controls eye movement, social behaviour, action planning and fine movement. The dominant frontal lobe acts together with the dominant temporal lobe to control speech production. The dominant lobe is that in the hemisphere which controls the preferred hand.
c. The outside of the temporal lobe acts together with the dominant parietal lobe to control speech input while the inside acts together with the dominant frontal lobe to control speech output.
d. The parietal lobe controls sensation and spatial orientation. Together with the temporal lobe they deal with the comprehension of speech and the so-called 'internal dialogue'. The latter is the 'voice inside the head' which develops in childhood and helps with working memory, in particular for creative persons, acting as a conversation with an imaginary audience.
e. The occipital lobe deals with vision.
f. The amygdala is a subcortical region connected with emotional responses and learning. It is part of the limbic system.
g. The hippocampus is a cortical region within the limbic system involved in memory formation and spatial navigation.
h. The thalamus is a mass of grey matter at the centre of the brain and is regarded as the gateway to the cortex, acting as a relay station of sensory impulses to the cortex.

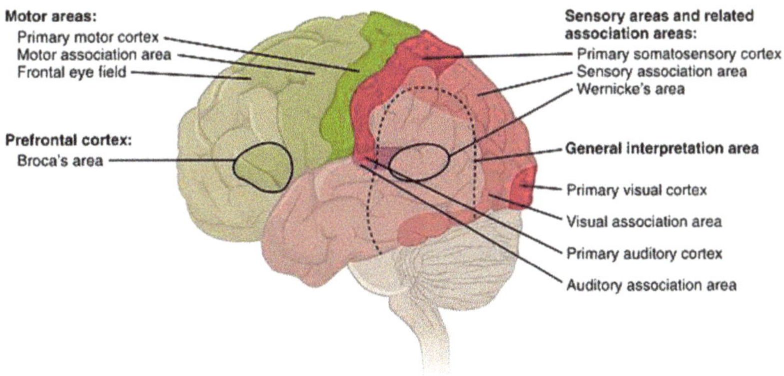

Figure 1.2. Key areas of the cerebral cortex (simplified left hemisphere) [3]. *Source*: OpenStax College https://commons.wikimedia.org/wiki/File:1604_Types_of_Cortical_Areas-02.jpg CC BY-SA 3.0.

i. The hypothalamus is responsible for maintaining a constant internal environment. It regulates basic desires such as hunger and thirst and coordinates the activities of the endocrine and autonomic nervous system.
j. The cerebral cortex is the outer layer of the cerebrum.

1.3 The cerebral cortex

The higher-level information-processing parts of the brain are in the *neocortex* [2]. It makes up most of the *cerebral cortex* and includes all the major sensory, motor, and association areas. Some key cortical features are shown in figure 1.2. The neocortex is composed of six laminated layers which are identifiable in a human adult. The second major type of cortex is the *allocortex*. It is thinner and contains three layers and includes the hippocampus (archicortex) and primary olfactory areas (paleocortex). The transitional zone between the neocortex and the allocortex is the *mesocortex*; it has between three and six layers and contains the cingulate and parahippocampal gyri. The non-neocortical areas have visceral and emotional roles and are mostly contained within the limbic lobe or primary olfactory areas. Broca's area has been traditionally thought to deal with speech production and Wernicke's area with the comprehension of speech. In fact, the sharp distinction between the production and comprehension of speech and language has recently been abandoned in favour of a more integrated function.

1.4 The electronic nature of the brain

To study the nervous system electronic engineers follow their philosophy of devising a *model* in electronic form. Thus we start with the *basic functional and structural building block*. This is taken to be the *neuron*, the nerve cell shown in figure 1.3 with its general features. Neurons communicate with each other with muscle fibres and with glands at *synapses*. The interconnection of these neurons results in a *neural network*. Then we attempt a description of a single neuron at key points, e.g. the

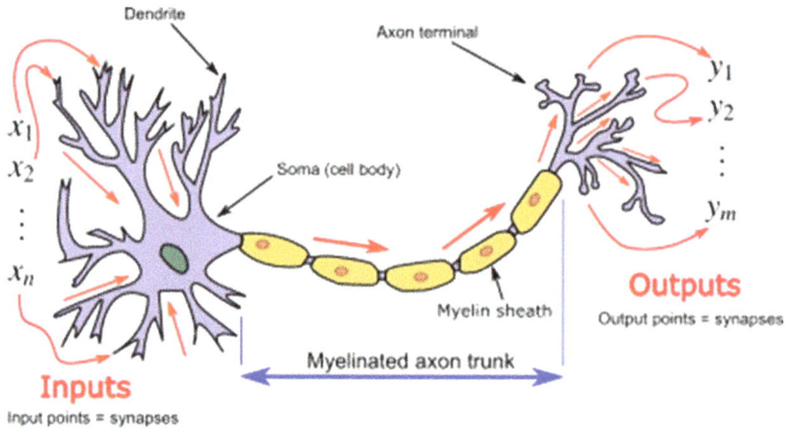

Figure 1.3. The basic elements of a neuron [4]. *Source*: Egm4313.s12 https://commons.wikimedia.org/wiki/File:Neuron3.png CC BY-SA 3.0.

input and output along its length, etc, in electronic terms. Next we determine the main properties of the arbitrary interconnection of these building blocks, again at points of interest. This is usually a circuit diagram which is called an *electronic network*. Then we say that this is an *electronic model* of the original biological neural network. In all cases, however, this is a very approximate model and can only serve as a starting point for a more comprehensive view of the nervous system.

Structurally, there are two main types of cortical neuron [3]. These are (i) granular neurons which are small cells common in sensory areas and (ii) pyramidal neurons which are large cells prominent in motor areas. The cerebral cortex also contains *Purkinje* cells which are similar to pyramidal neurons.

In terms of their function, neurons are of three types:

i. Afferent neurons carrying signals towards the brain or central nervous system (CNS); sensory neurons satisfy this definition.
ii. Efferent neurons carrying signals away from the brain or CNS; motor neurons satisfy this definition.
iii. Association (interneurons) transforming sensory excitations into motor responses.

In all its guises, the neuron has the same basic functional structure shown in figure 1.3 composed of dendrites, a cell body, an axon, and axon terminals.

The mechanism of conduction of signals in the brain and nervous system is now explained briefly with reference to figures 1.3 and 1.4. A neuron has a *resting* voltage (potential difference) of −70 mV between its interior and exterior. This is a result of the presence of ions (notably sodium and potassium ions) in the vicinity of the cell membrane made of a bilayer, the inside of which acts like a dielectric (insulator). An atom of matter has an equal number of electrons (negative charges) and protons (positive charges) and hence it is electrically neutral. If it loses an electron it becomes a positive ion and if it gains an electron it becomes a negative ion. The same applies

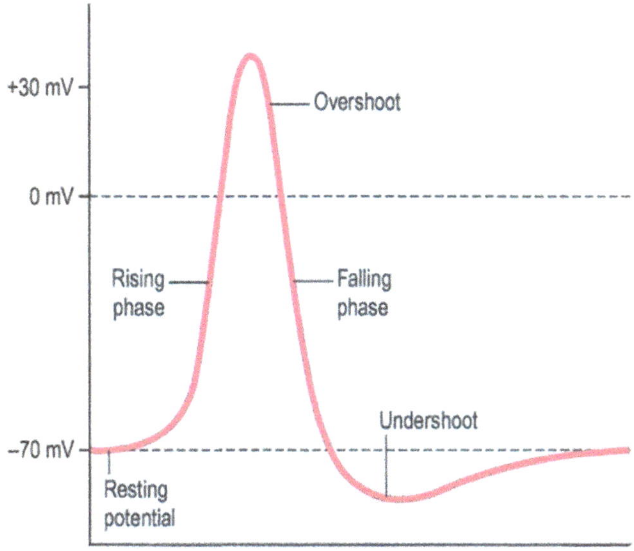

Figure 1.4. Action potential.

to molecules. The diffusion of ions across the membrane and the electrostatic forces (see the next section) reach an equilibrium forming the resting potential. Excitation from other neurons changes the membrane voltage until it reaches a threshold then it creates an *action potential* forming a pulse of a about +40 mV with a few milliseconds (ms) duration which has the general appearance shown in figure 1.4. This propagates as a state of depolarisation from section to section along the axon until it reaches a *synapse* where the neurotransmitter, a biochemical compound, connects the axon to the dendrite of another neuron. The speed of propagation is aided by the insulator *myelin sheath* composed of a series of sections within which the impulses are transmitted. This myelin wrapping is a lipid-rich sheath containing oligodendrocytes and peripheral Schwann cells [2]. It increases the axonal conduction velocity. Generation of the signals also takes place at the junctions between the sections known as *nodes of Ranvier* at which there are many ion channels. This process is called *saltatory conduction.* Provided the pulse satisfies certain conditions, it is transferred to the receiving neuron and alters its membrane voltage. This gives rise to either an excitory or inhibitory response and is the signalling mechanism in the nervous system.

Unlike digital computers, in which processing and storage are performed separately, both tasks are intertwined in the brain using about 10^{11} neurons and 10^{14} synapses. Therefore, a good simulation of the brain must ideally model this attribute, resulting in a so-called *neuromorphic* model.

Another major difference between the brain and a digital computer is that, in the latter, the processing requires a central synchronising clock while the brain achieves all the processing without a clock, despite the fact that self-synchronisation is definitely present in the brain by means of brain waves which are by-products of neural networks.

The analogy with a digital computer model is inaccurate. A better idea is to speak of a *signal processing* system. An interesting outcome of this is that when neuroscientists examine the complex interconnection of neurons, they arrive at a system which does more complex tasks than what they can infer from the properties of the simple building blocks, so much so that they feel compelled to give this property a new name—an *emergent property*. For electronic engineers this is hardly surprising at all since this is precisely what they do in every design, namely achieve greater complexity from very simple components, and they do not need to give a new name to this property—it is simply an inherent characteristic of the design process.

1.5 Modelling biological systems by electronic circuits

Modelling biological systems using electronic systems has been extremely successful. An example which has a significant neurological content is shown in figure 1.5 and includes the cochlea [5] (the spiral part of the human ear that is the seat of hearing). Sound is directed by the pinna into the ear canal where, as it passes, it can

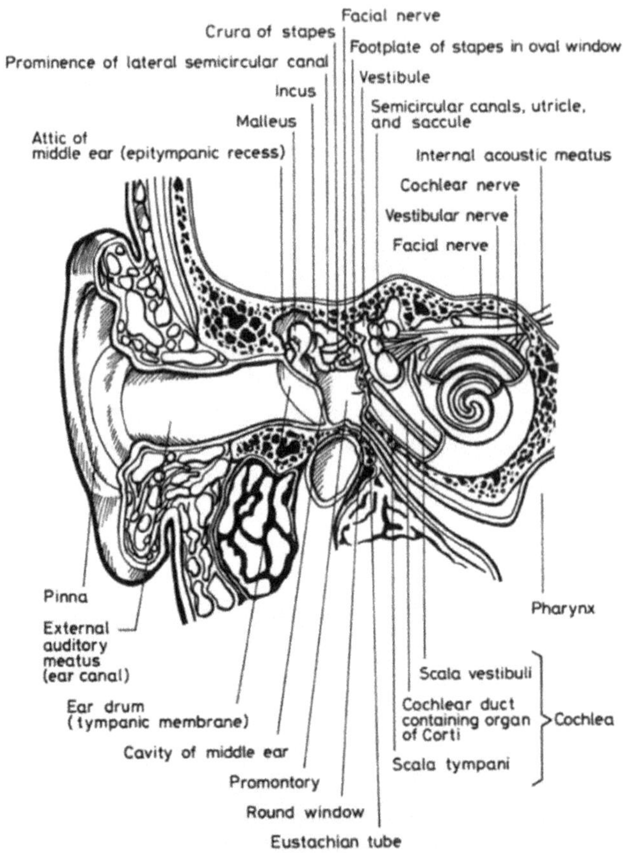

Figure 1.5. Illustration including the human cochlea. Reproduced with permission from [5]. Copyright 1990 Wiley.

be viewed as a plane wave relative to the small diameter of the ear canal (a spherical wave is perceived as a plane wave if the size of the receiver is very small compared with the diameter of the sphere). Most of the energy delivered to the ear drum is absorbed. The sound is transmitted to the cochlea (inner ear) via the ossicles which are the malleus, the incus and the stapes. The motion of the stapes displaces the fluid in the upper chamber of the cochlea. An equal amount of fluid is displaced at the round window since the net volume of the fluid within the cochlea must remain constant.

Figure 1.6 shows a rudimentary electronic network model which was proposed a long time ago to characterise the stapes, annular ligament, and cochlea [5]. This model can also be applied to the system which includes the entire middle ear and the ear drum. The annular ligament is represented by the non-linear capacitor C_{al} while the mass of the ossicles are represented by the inductor L_V. L_s is the mass of fluid behind the stapes while the elements between the nodes P_v and P_{rw} represent the behaviour of the cochlea. C_{rw} represents the stiffness of the round window. In this model, the one-to-one correspondence between the mechanical (physical) and electrical properties relies on the equivalence of (i) friction to resistance, (ii) mass to inductance, and (iii) stiffness to capacitance. This is based on energy considerations: (i) both friction and resistance *dissipate* (lose) energy; (ii) both mass and

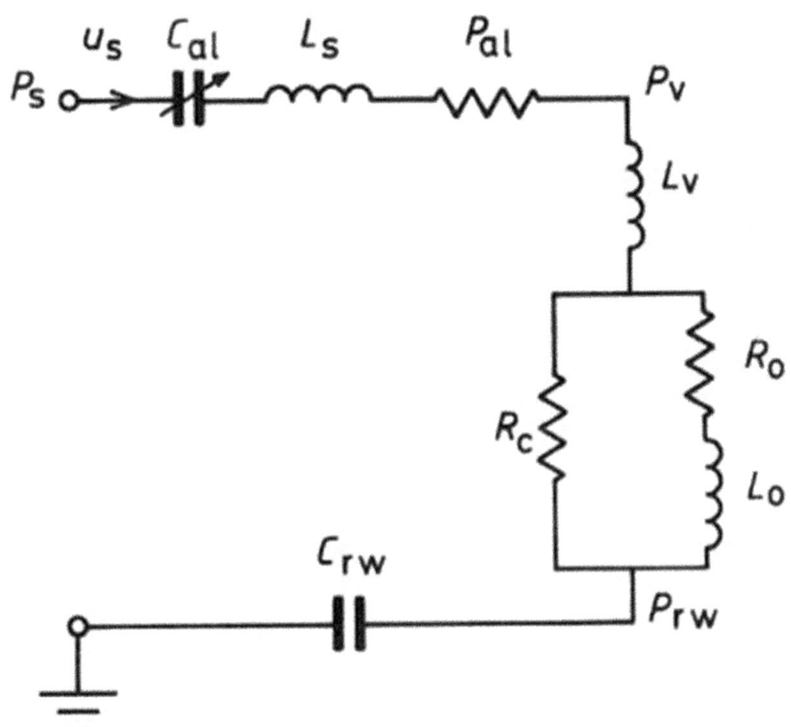

Figure 1.6. Electronic circuit model of the stapes, annular ligament, and cochlea.Reproduced with permission from [5]. Copyright 1990 Wiley.

inductance *store* analogous types of energy; while (iii) stiffness and capacitance *store* analogous types of energy. In this example it is possible for the model to be composed of passive components only. In other cases, one might require active components (e.g. transistors and electronic voltage and current sources).

This example has been given only as an illustration of the methodology of *modelling* which is inherent in the discipline of electronic engineering. It is a very powerful approach because we can use the electronic model to study the biological system in a non-invasive manner and modify the model without affecting the biological organism to which it belongs. The wealth of methods of electronic engineering which rely on the accumulated mathematical and circuit design knowledge can be used to huge advantage. One can increase the complexity of the model in accordance with the complexity of the biological system by successive approximation until ideally, but unattainably, an electronic copy of the biological system is achieved. A bionic version! But this is the subject of bio-inspired electronics which is another story.

1.6 The logic of synthesis [6]

The reasoning employed in the above example is inherent in the idea of modelling. One seeks a one-to-one correspondence between a biological unit and an equivalent electrical building block with analogous characteristics. Then the electronic model is constructed. This procedure highlights the distinctive nature of electronic engineering as a discipline relying on *synthesis* of ideas and components whereas many other disciplines are *analytical*. For example, in biology we are presented with a complete working system and we are required to reduce it to its constituent parts—this is *analysis*. In engineering, the opposite takes place in the *creative process of design* which requires that we start with basic building blocks and synthesise them to form a whole to perform a certain well-defined task or meet a set of specifications. Having designed and built the system, *analysis* can be performed to test the system performance and check whether it meets the specifications.

At the heart of signalling and communication in the nervous system there are three areas of electronic engineering, namely electric field theory, microelectronic circuits, and spectral analysis. We give an outline of the first two of these in the next sections, while the third is treated in later chapters.

1.7 Electric field theory

As employed in science and engineering, the term *field* is meant to describe a region where any type of force exists. The force can have many varied origins such as electric, magnetic, or gravitational, but ultimately it is helpful to visualise the force as having a mechanical *effect*, i.e. it can move an object if the object is allowed to move.

Fields can be static or time varying. A basic law of electrostatics (static electric fields) is *Coulomb's law*. It states that 'The force between two small charges Q_1 and Q_2 separated in a uniform homogeneous medium by a distance r, which is large compared with their linear dimensions, is directly proportional to the product of the charges and inversely proportional to the square of the distance between them. The direction of the force is along the line joining the charges':

$$F \propto \frac{Q_1 Q_2}{r^2}$$

$$\therefore F = k\frac{Q_1 Q_2}{r^2}$$

$$k = 1/4\pi\varepsilon.$$

ε is called the permittivity of the medium in which the charges are placed:

$\varepsilon = \varepsilon_0 \varepsilon_r$

$\varepsilon_0 = 1/(36\pi \times 10^9) = 8.85 \times 10^{-12}$ farads m^{-1} (Fm^{-1})

ε_r = relative permittivity (dimensionless).

Q_1 and Q_2 are in coulombs (C), r is in metres (m), F is in newtons (N).

We use an arrow on a symbol to denote a vector, i.e. a quantity that is defined by a magnitude and a direction. Normal symbols denote scalars—quantities that require only a magnitude for their complete definition. The forces being vectors, we should write

$$\vec{F} = \frac{Q_1 Q_2}{4\pi\varepsilon r^2}\vec{a}_r,$$

where $\vec{a}_r$ is a unit vector in the direction of r.

The presence of an *electric field* in a given region can be detected by bringing into that region a test charge, i.e. a small positively charged body, and determining whether a force is exerted on this test charge. If such a force exists, we say that an electric field is present. Note that when we say *force*, we mean a mechanical force of electric origin. In other words the body will *tend to move* if allowed. The electric field intensity $\vec{E}$ at any point is therefore defined as the force on a unit positive charge placed at the at point, i.e. it is the force per unit charge:

$$\vec{E} = \frac{Q}{4\pi\varepsilon r^2}\vec{a}_r.$$

The potential difference between two points A and B in an electric field $\vec{E}$ is defined as the external work done in moving a unit positive charge from point B to point A. B is the initial position and A is the final position:

$$W = \int_{\text{initial}}^{\text{final}} \vec{F} \cdot \mathrm{d}\vec{L}$$

$$V_{AB} = -\int_{B}^{A} \vec{E} \cdot \mathrm{d}\vec{L}.$$

The term inside the integral is the *scalar* or *dot* product of the two vectors. It is a scalar of value equalling the product if the two magnitudes multiplied by the cosine of the angle between the two vectors.

For a point charge

$$V_{AB} = -\frac{Q}{4\pi\varepsilon}\int_{r_B}^{r_A} \frac{dr}{r^2}$$

$$= \frac{Q}{4\pi\varepsilon}\left[\frac{1}{r_A} - \frac{1}{r_B}\right]$$

$$\therefore \oint \vec{E}\cdot d\vec{L} = 0,$$

with $r_B \rightarrow \infty$ so that

$$V_{AB} = V_A = \frac{Q}{4\pi\varepsilon}\frac{1}{r_A}.$$

V_A is called the absolute potential of the point A, i.e. the potential with respect to infinity.

Charges can be distributed over a surface with uniform density in C m^{-2} or over a volume with a volume density in C m^{-3} or over a line with linear density in C m^{-1}. In its most general form, the electric field is the gradient of the electric potential, with

$$\nabla = \left(\frac{\partial}{\partial x}\vec{a}_x + \frac{\partial}{\partial y}\vec{a}_y + \frac{\partial}{\partial z}\vec{a}_z\right)$$

$$\vec{E}(x, y, z, t) = -\nabla V(x, y, z, t),$$

where t is the time variable and the a's are unit vectors in the directions of the three coordinates x, y, and z respectively, in the Cartesian system. This relationship means that the electric field is a vector whose components in the three dimensions are the rates of change of the electric potential (voltage) in the three directions. This is true whether the voltage is static or time varying. The electric flux density measures the number of flux lines per unit area and is given by the vector

$$\vec{D} = \varepsilon\vec{E}.$$

1.7.1 Capacitance

The capacitance C between two electrodes a and b is a measure of the charge Q on each electrode per volt of potential difference ($V_a - V_b$):

$$C = \frac{Q}{V_a - V_b}.$$

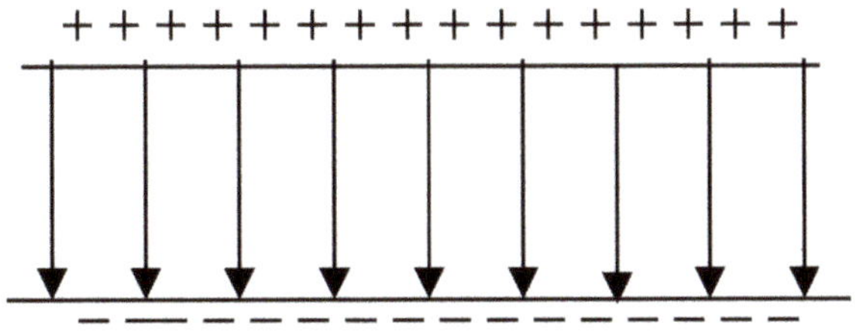

Figure 1.7. A parallel plate capacitor.

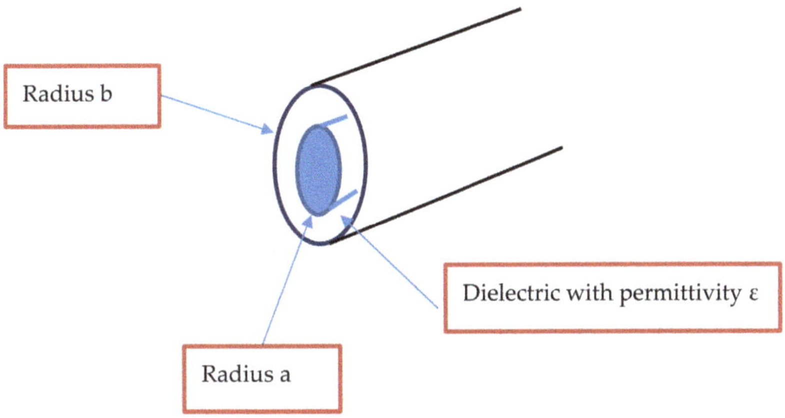

Figure 1.8. Concentric cylinders.

For example, in the case of parallel plates as shown in figure 1.7, the charge density on each plate is σ. Since $\vec{E} = \vec{D}/\varepsilon$ is assumed uniform,

$$V_a - V_b = E \cdot d = \sigma d/\varepsilon.$$

The total charge on each plate of area A is σA:

$$\therefore C = \frac{\sigma A}{V_a - V_b} = \frac{\varepsilon A}{d}\ \mathrm{F},$$

where F stands for Farad. Similar calculations for concentric cylinders as shown in figure 1.8 give the capacitance per metre as

$$C = 2\pi\varepsilon/\ln(b/a)\ \mathrm{F\ m^{-1}}.$$

This expression can be useful when attempting to model neurons as RC ladder networks.

1.7.2 Electric current and current density

When an electric field $\vec{E}$ is applied to a conductor in a given direction, the free or conduction electrons (valence electrons) of the constituent atoms acquire an average drift velocity $\vec{u}$ in the direction opposite to that of the electric field. The concepts of current and current density are introduced to describe the flow of charges. The conduction current density is defined by a vector $\vec{J_c}$ having the direction of flow of charges and a magnitude equal to the number of charges per second which cross a unit area perpendicular to the direction of flow.

If n is the number of free charges per m^3, then

$$\vec{J_c} = nq\vec{u} \quad \left[\frac{C}{m^3} \cdot \frac{m}{s}\right] = [A/m^2].$$

The conduction current is defined as the rate at which charges pass through any given surface area and is, therefore, a scalar quantity since charges can cross a surface in any direction. If the current density at any point on the surface is $\vec{J_c}$, then the total current through the surface is

$$I_c = \int_S \vec{J_c} \cdot d\vec{S}.$$

1.7.3 Displacement current

This is an unusual kind of current in contrast with the more familiar conduction current. It is necessary for the interrelationship between electric and magnetic fields. Consider a closed surface S enclosing a volume V with current i_1 entering and current i_2 leaving it as shown in figure 1.9.

If i_1 is different from i_2, this means that there is either an accumulation of charges within the volume (if $i_1 > i_2$) or a decrease of the charges originally present within the volume (if $i_1 < i_2$). Thus

$$i_1 - i_2 = \frac{dq}{dt}.$$

Gauss's law equates the electric flux (flow) through any closed surface to the charge enclosed by the surface. If D denotes the charge density over the surface, then

$$\psi = q = \oint_S \vec{D} \cdot d\vec{S},$$

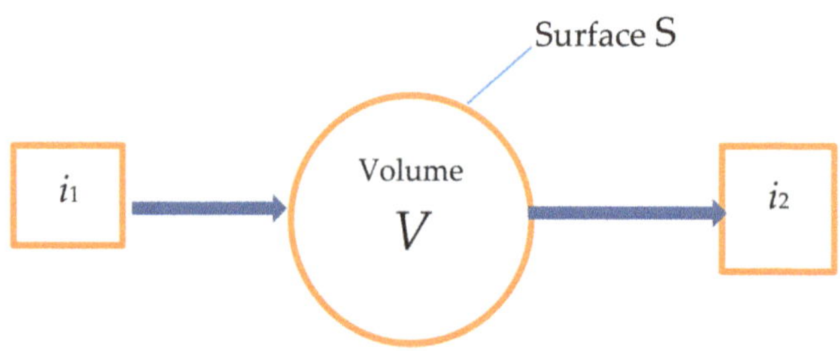

Figure 1.9. Pertinent to the concept of displacement current.

So that the time rate of change of charge becomes the current and we have

$$i_1 - i_2 = \frac{\mathrm{d}\psi}{\mathrm{d}t}$$

$$i_1 = i_2 + \frac{\mathrm{d}\psi}{\mathrm{d}t}.$$

The rate of change of flux $\frac{\mathrm{d}\psi}{\mathrm{d}t}$ is called the *displacement current*. Thus we conclude that the total current entering any volume is equal to the total current leaving the volume provided the displacement current is added to the conduction current. This is a more general statement of the familiar Kirchhoff's law which states that the current entering a node in an electric circuit equals the current leaving the node. The displacement current is

$$\vec{i}_{\mathrm{d}} = \frac{\partial\psi}{\partial t} = \frac{\partial}{\partial t}\oint_S \vec{D}\cdot \mathrm{d}\vec{S} = \oint_S \frac{\partial\vec{D}}{\partial t}\cdot \mathrm{d}\vec{S}$$

and we define displacement current density as

$$\vec{J}_{\mathrm{d}} = \frac{\partial\vec{D}}{\partial t}.$$

We also have Ohm's law governing the conduction current for a current carrying conductor:

$$V = IR$$

$$R = \frac{\text{resistivity} \times \text{length}}{\text{area}}$$

$$= \frac{\text{length}}{\text{conductivity} \times \text{area}},$$

which leads to the conduction current density (current per unit area)

$$\vec{J}_{\mathrm{c}} = \sigma_{\mathrm{c}} \cdot \vec{E},$$

with

$$\sigma_{\mathrm{c}} = \frac{nqu}{E} = nq\mu^{\pm}$$

$$\mu = \frac{u}{E},$$

where n is the number of charge carriers per unit volume, q is the value of the charge causing the conduction, σ_{c} is the conductivity of the material, and μ is called the *mobility* of the charges, i.e. it is the velocity per unit of electric field.

1.8 MOS transistors and microelectronic circuits [7, 8]

Now, just as we defined a basic building block of the nervous system, it is appropriate to decide on a basic building block for the electronic system which will be used to model the brain. The basic building block of most electronic integrated circuits is the metal oxide semiconductor (MOS) transistor shown in figure 1.10 with its symbols in figure 1.11. It consists of three types of material: (i) a metal which is a conductor used as electrodes connecting the device to other components; (ii) an oxide which is an insulator; and (iii) a semiconductor of n- or p-type which can be silicon, whose electrical properties lie between those of insulators and conductors.

Conductors are simply materials which have a very large number of mobile electrons which can be freed easily from their atoms because they are loosely bound to them. Their movement can be accelerated by applying an electric voltage resulting in an electric field; the higher it is the faster the flow of electrons, which is defined as an electric current. In other words, a conductor has high a mobility value. The ratio

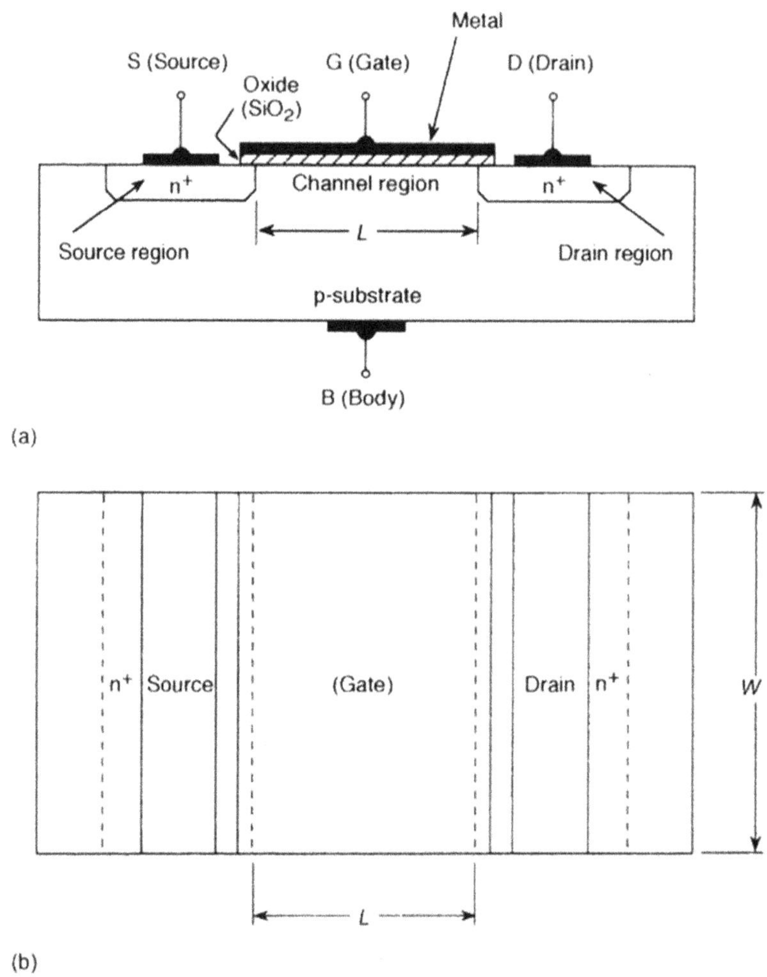

Figure 1.10. The enhancement-type MOSFET: (a) cross-section and (b) top view.

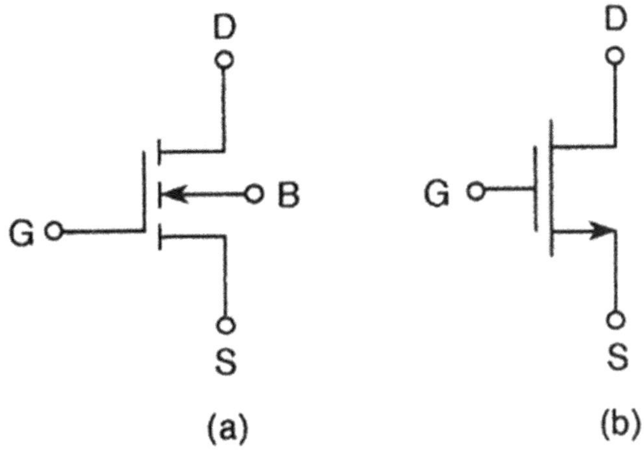

Figure 1.11. Symbols of the NMOSFET: (a) showing the substrate and (b) simplified symbols when B is connected to S.

of the voltage to the current defines the resistance of the conductor. The resistance of a length of wire of length l and uniform cross-sectional area A is

$$R = \frac{l}{\sigma A}\ \Omega\ \text{(ohms)},$$

where σ is called the conductivity of the material and is very high for a good conductor. The relation between the voltage $v(t)$ across a resistor and its current $i(t)$ is given by

$$v(t) = Ri(t).$$

On the other hand, an insulator has very few free electrons because the outer shell electrons are tightly bound to the nucleus, and one would need very large voltages to free them, and if this happens the insulation breaks down and collapses and the device would be of no use as an insulator. In other words, an insulator has a very low mobility value. The conductivity of a good insulator is very low. If we have a piece of insulator of thickness d and uniform cross-sectional area A and insert it between two conductors (electrodes) we form a capacitor. The value of the capacitance will be

$$C = \frac{\varepsilon A}{d}\ \text{F (farads)},$$

where ε is called the permittivity of the material. If a voltage difference $v(t)$ is applied across the capacitor, a charge accumulates of value $q(t) = \pm C\ v(t)$ and a current results of value

$$i(t) = -C\frac{\mathrm{d}v(t)}{\mathrm{d}t}\ \text{A (amperes)}$$

and if the voltage is static V, then there is simply a charge Q of value $\pm CV$ on the plates (electrodes) of the capacitor.

Now, if we take a piece of a certain kind of semiconductor and apply a voltage across it, we create an electric field according to the definition given earlier. At a certain temperature some of the electrons in the outer shells of the atoms leave and migrate moving in a direction opposite to that of the electric field because they are negatively charged particles. This creates an electric current which is defined as the motion of charges. Another type of semiconductor is such that the majority charge carriers are atoms which have a shortage of electrons and as far as charges are concerned, they are positively charged, and they behave like *holes*. The first type is called an *n-type* while the second is a *p-type*. In either case, the material has an intermediate mobility of the charge carriers between that of a conductor and that of an insulator. Very often we add dopants in each type to increase the number of charge carriers and we speak of n^+ and p^+ materials. This combination of n-type and p-type semiconductors are used to fabricate junctions across which electrons and holes flow in opposite directions creating current in a controlled manner. Thus, a whole family of semiconductor devices can be created which include diodes and transistors. We can calculate the current due to electrons and holes crossing *pn-junctions* using quantum mechanics.

The MOS device is fabricated by a special process which results in one of the most versatile and useful building blocks of electronic engineering. Huge numbers of this transistor, reaching hundreds of millions, can be manufactured and placed on a single small *microchip* to perform complex tasks with lightning speeds. We can place entire electronic systems on a single chip, which has resulted in the new design of the *system on a chip* (*SOC*). The transistor itself has several regions or *modes* of operation depending on the choice of operating range of voltages and currents. The device is accessible via four electrodes connected to the various regions. These are called the *source*, *gate*, *drain*, and *substrate*. The input to the device is usually between the gate and the source while the substrate is also very often connected to the source. To prepare the device for operation it must be *biased*. This means that we connect dc voltages to some of the terminals such that we determine the nature of the device in terms of its function. There is a *threshold voltage* below which the device will not conduct electrical current in the conventional sense. The biasing conditions are set to place the operating conditions within a specific range which determines the application in which the device may be used. We have a number of possibilities which include:

a. An amplifying device used for the design of analog circuits.
b. A simple ON/OFF switch which is the basic device in digital circuits and digital computers.
c. If it is operated in the subthreshold region, it can simulate the behaviour of a neuron in an approximate but instructive manner. This is a *happy accident* for both electronic engineers and neuroscientists, or perhaps a gift from Mother Nature.

1.9 Conclusion

An electronic engineering perspective of the brain is both appropriate and instructive. It has led to a deep understanding of the brain function and yielded many diagnostic and treatment tools without which modern neuromedicine would not be possible. It is unfortunate that the basic techniques of electronic engineering do not form part of the education of health care professionals. This chapter has provided some useful material and directions in this regard. The rest of the book continues along similar lines.

References

[1] National Institute on Aging 2008 File:Side View of the Brain.png *Wikimedia Commons* https://commons.wikimedia.org/wiki/File:Side_View_of_the_Brain.png

[2] Johns P 2014 *Clinical Neuroscience* (London: Churchill Livingstone Elsevier)

[3] OpenStax College 2013 File:1604 Types of Cortical Areas-02.jpg *Wikimedia Commons* https://commons.wikimedia.org/wiki/File:1604_Types_of_Cortical_Areas-02.jpg

[4] Egm4313.s12 2018 File:Neuron3.png *Wikimedia Commons* https://commons.wikimedia.org/wiki/File:Neuron3.png

[5] Baher H 1990 *Analog and Digital Signal Processing* (New York: Wiley)

[6] Baher H 1984 *Synthesis of Electrical Networks* (New York: Wiley)

[7] Baher H 2012 *Signal Processing and Integrated Circuits* (New York: Wiley)

[8] Baher H 1996 *Microelectronic Switched Capacitor Filters* (New York: Wiley)

IOP Publishing

Electronic Engineering for Neuromedicine

Hussein Baher

Chapter 2

The brain as a signal processor

2.1 Introduction

In this chapter the brain is introduced as an electronic signal processing system and the basic differences between the human brain and man-made digital information processing systems are emphasised and highlighted. Methods for modelling neurons, and hence the brain, using the tools of electronic engineering are introduced in their elementary forms. Also, we discuss the number of ways in which the brain signals are accessed and outline the techniques of the analysis and processing of such signals.

2.2 Signals and systems [1, 2]

A *signal* is a physical quality or quantity which conveys information. Figure 2.1 shows examples of signals as functions of time. A system is a collection of components which accepts signals and produces output(s) different from the input (s) according to certain rules; in other words the system *processes* the signals.

Signals can be natural or man-made. Either type can also be deterministic or random. The brain is constantly sending signals to various parts of the body which cause them to perform certain tasks or react in particular ways. Therefore, the brain signal is called an *excitation* and the action performed by the particular organ is called a *response*. These signals also propagate within the brain. In either case, signals are transmitted from one point to another for the purpose of conveying information. The signals we deal with are of two main types—purely electrical and electrochemical—although the latter can be ultimately viewed as electrical. So, we characterise the signals by voltages and currents. This is the nature of the information-carrying and processing of signals of the brain. Hence, we view the parts of the brain we happen to describe as *signal processing systems.*

2.3 Spectrum analysis [2]

A continuous time signal is defined for all values of time. A discrete-time signal is defined only for discrete values of time. If the amplitudes of the signal are also

doi:10.1088/978-0-7503-3427-3ch2

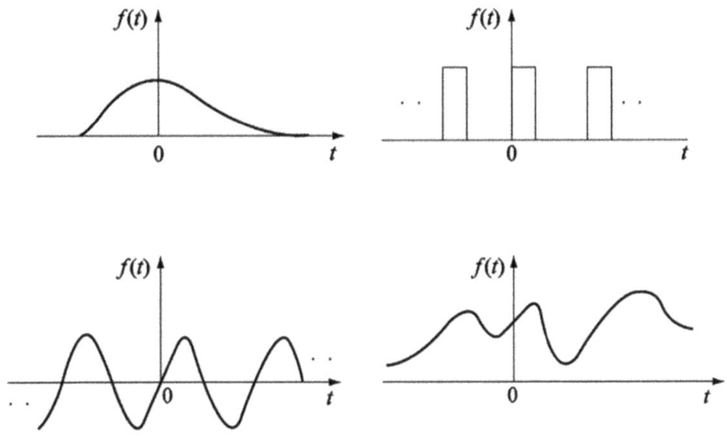

Figure 2.1. Examples of time signals.

discrete and encoded, then the signal is in digital form. In a certain approach, the discrete spikes are coded by their network location and time. This is highly original since time and location are extremely important in the brain. Also, some processing is done in analog form by charge accumulation, whereas the transmission or communication is performed by pulses which are discrete-time signals akin to digital signals. Therefore brain signals are always analog, but a mixture of continuous and discrete in time. The mathematical techniques for dealing with discrete signals are the same as those used for digital signals. Nevertheless, the brain is an analog system processing analog signals even if they are of the discrete-time type. Remember, a 'digital' brain would need converters to interface with the analog world we live in.

The observation of signals in real time has its limitations when dealing with complex signals. More appropriate methods for the analysis of signals rely on the conversion of a signal into its frequency-domain representation. The information about the signal is exactly the same and completely preserved but much clearer for highly complex signals. A sine wave for example becomes a single vertical line at the frequency of the wave. For more complex signals we need *spectral analysis* relying on the *Fourier transform*.

The Fourier transform of a signal $f(t)$ as a function of time t gives the frequency-domain representation of the signal. This relation between the time-domain and frequency-domain representations is given by the expressions

$$F(\omega) = \int_{-\infty}^{\infty} f(t)\exp(-\mathrm{j}\omega t)\,\mathrm{d}t,$$

in which ω is the radian frequency in radians per second, which is $2\pi \times$ the frequency in Hz, and

$$f(t) = \frac{1}{2\pi}\int_{-\infty}^{\infty} F(\omega)\exp(\mathrm{j}\omega t)\,\mathrm{d}\omega$$

$$F(\omega) = \Im[f(t)]$$

$$f(t) = \Im^{-1}[F(\omega)],$$

and the notation

$$f(t) \leftrightarrow F(\omega)$$

is used to signify that $f(t)$ and $F(\omega)$ form a *Fourier transform pair*.

The Fourier transform $F(\omega)$ of $f(t)$ is a *complex* function of ω, so that we may write

$$F(\omega) = |F(\omega)| \exp(j\varphi(\omega)),$$

where ω is a continuous frequency variable. This means that a plot of $|F(\omega)|$ against ω now gives the (continuous) *amplitude spectrum* of $f(t)$, while $\varphi(\omega)$ plotted against ω gives the (continuous) *phase spectrum* of $f(t)$. An example is shown in figure 2.2.

The Fourier transform of a periodic function with a period $T = 2\pi/\omega_0$ is an infinite train of equidistant impulses as expressed in

$$F_p(\omega) = \omega_0 \sum_{k=-\infty}^{\infty} F(k\omega_0)\delta(\omega - k\omega_0),$$

where $F(k\omega_0)$ is the Fourier transform of $f(t)$ evaluated at the discrete set of frequencies $k\omega_0$, i.e.

$$F(k\omega_0) = \int_{-T/2}^{T/2} f(t)\exp(-jk\omega_0 t)\,dt.$$

Figure 2.3 shows an example of a periodic signal with its spectrum. The spectrum contains all the information as the time-domain representation.

For periodic signals, a convenient way is to represent the signal as the infinite sum of pure sine and cosine waves as

$$f(t) = \frac{a_0}{2} + \sum_{k=1}^{\infty}(a_k \cos k\omega_0 t + b_k \sin k\omega_0 t)$$

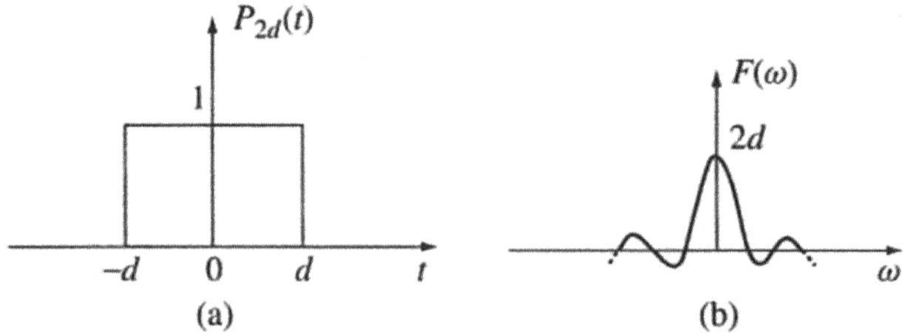

Figure 2.2. (a) A pulse and (b) its spectrum.

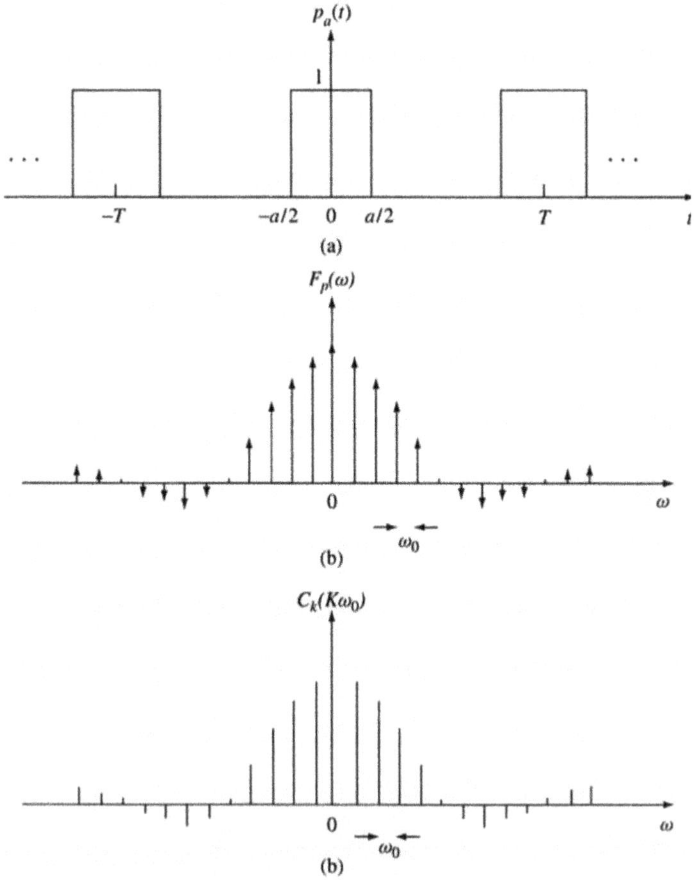

Figure 2.3. (a) A periodic train of rectangular pulses, (b) its spectrum as a train of impulses, and (c) its spectrum as a plot of the spectral lines, which are the magnitudes of the Fourier series coefficients.

$$a_k = \frac{2}{T}\int_{-T/2}^{T/2} f(t)\cos k\omega_0 t \, \mathrm{d}t$$

$$b_k = \frac{2}{T}\int_{-T/2}^{T/2} f(t)\sin k\omega_0 t \, \mathrm{d}t$$

$$\omega_0 = 2\pi/T,$$

with T being the *period* and ω_0 the fundamental radian frequency.

Parseval's theorem relates the *average power* of a signal to the *sum of the squares* of the amplitudes of the complex Fourier coefficients as expressed by

$$\sum_{k=-\infty}^{\infty} |c_k|^2 = \frac{1}{T}\int_{-T/2}^{T/2} [f(t)]^2 \mathrm{d}t.$$

The squared amplitudes of the complex Fourier coefficients are called the *power spectral amplitudes* and a plot of these versus frequency is called the *power spectrum* of the signal.

The *energy spectral density* (or *energy spectrum*) of a signal is the square of the modulus of its Fourier transform

$$E(\omega) \triangleq \left|F(\omega)\right|^2$$

so that

$$W = \frac{1}{2\pi}\int_{-\infty}^{\infty} E(\omega)\,\mathrm{d}\omega = \int_{-\infty}^{\infty} |f(t)|^2\,\mathrm{d}t.$$

This is Parseval's theorem, which highlights the fact that the energy in the spectrum equals the energy in the parent signal of time. Such signals are called *finite-energy* signals.

In neural signal processing, the signals are often displayed in the frequency domain and their spectra are analysed and examined for the relevant information. The instruments used are called *spectrum analysers*, which incorporate software tools called *fast Fourier transform* (FFT) algorithms. These are high-speed mathematical algorithms used to calculate the Fourier transforms of the signals, hence their spectra, which are then displayed on screens for examination.

2.3.1 Correlation functions

The *autocorrelation* of a signal is defined by

$$\rho_{ff}(\tau) = \int_{-\infty}^{\infty} f(t)f(t+\tau)\,\mathrm{d}\tau.$$

For a finite-energy signal, the *autocorrelation* and the *energy spectrum* form a Fourier transform pair

$$\rho_{ff}(\tau) \leftrightarrow E(\omega).$$

For two finite-energy signals, the *cross-correlation* is defined by

$$\rho_{fg}(\tau) = \int_{-\infty}^{\infty} f(t)g(t+\tau)\,\mathrm{d}t.$$

The *cross-energy spectrum* of the two signals is defined by

$$\Im\left[\rho_{fg}(\tau)\right] = F^*(\omega)G(\omega) = E_{fg}(\omega),$$

which is the Fourier transform of the cross-correlation, and this is a measure of the similarity between the two signals. The asterisk denotes the complex conjugate.

A *causal signal* is one that is zero for negative values of time. A *causal system* is a system whose impulse response is a causal signal.

The Fourier transform of a periodic train of impulses is another train of impulses as given by

$$\sum_{k=-\infty}^{\infty} \delta(t - kT) \leftrightarrow \omega_0 \sum_{k=-\infty}^{\infty} \delta(\omega - k\omega_0).$$

2.3.2 Periodic signals

The Fourier transform of a periodic function is an infinite train of equidistant impulses as expressed in

$$F_p(\omega) = \omega_0 \sum_{k=-\infty}^{\infty} F(k\omega_0)\delta(\omega - k\omega_0),$$

where $F(k\omega_0)$ is the Fourier transform of $f(t)$ evaluated at the discrete set of frequencies $k\omega_0$, i.e.

$$F(k\omega_0) = \int_{-T/2}^{T/2} f(t)\exp(-jk\omega_0 t)\,dt.$$

2.4 Modelling the brain

As pointed out before, there are basic differences between biological and artificial (man-made) information processing systems. Notably, human behaviour is goal-oriented using *inductive logic* to work successfully in nonlinear nonstationary non-Gaussian environment throughout the evolutionary path. On the other hand, man-made automata use sensors and computational algorithms which are generally still unable to match the biological information system but only capable of increasing the speeds and precision.

Digital computers have been with us for a long time. They have always relied on a very old architecture called the *von Neumann* machine. It has separate parts: one for computation and the other for memory and storage as shown in figure 2.4. This served us well when computers were considered merely glorified calculators doing arithmetic at very high speeds. More recently, as we demanded a higher degree of sophistication from computers, we began to see the drawbacks of this architecture, particularly when we started to design systems which may simulate the brain.

In a certain sense, all the inherent weaknesses of this aging inefficient system have been covered up by the increasing the number and speed of the transistors which can be put on a single integrated circuit.

To be able to simulate the human brain, the von Neumann architecture has to be abandoned and for a true neuromorphic (brain-like) electronic system a radical approach must be invented.

A very simple model of a neuron that may be used to explain some of its most basic properties, such as the action potential and signalling, is to use an RC ladder network, as shown in figure 2.5, which is basically a low-pass filter (passing low frequencies and attenuating higher frequencies) with the series resistance as the axial

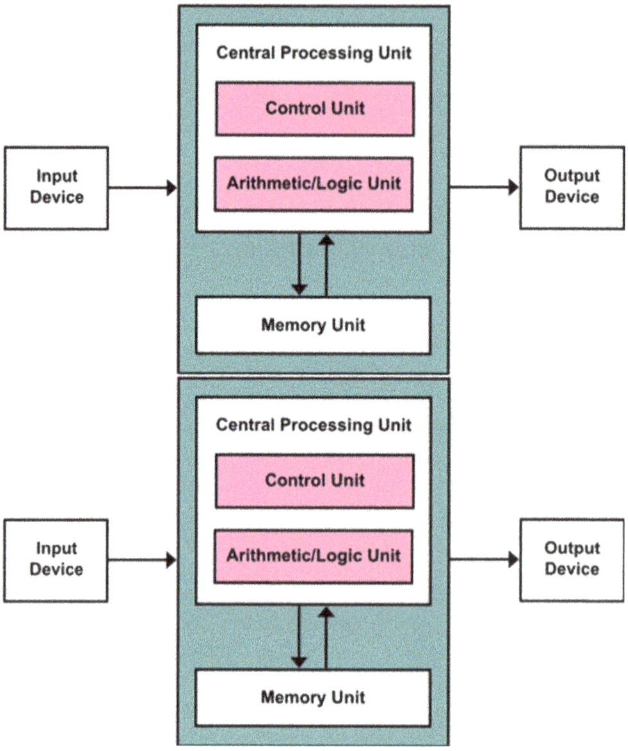

Figure 2.4. The so-called von Neumann architecture of conventional computers [4]. This is **not** how the human brain functions. *Source*: Kapooht https://commons.wikimedia.org/wiki/File:Von_Neumann_Architecture.svg CC BY-SA 3.0.

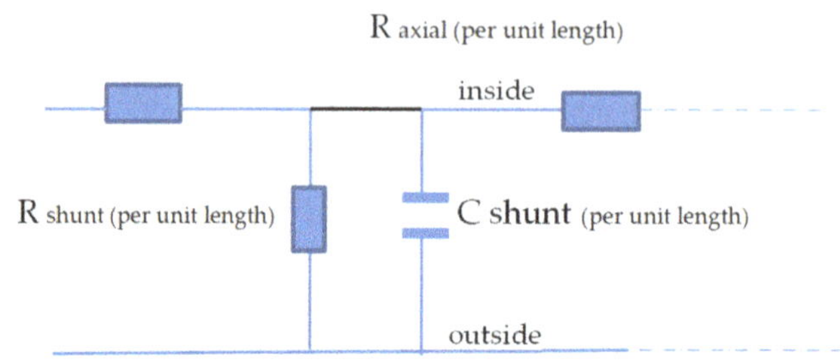

Figure 2.5. RC ladder network for modelling a neuron.

resistance along the axon and the shunt impedance as that between the outside and inside of the cell which has resistive and capacitive components. These are distributed uniformly along the axon. Analysis of this network is a simple and straightforward exercise for electronic engineers and the frequency response is used to examine the properties of the neuron. The calculation of the resistance and capacitance values follow the methods of electric fields and circuits given earlier.

A more accurate model would be as a distributed network composed of transmission lines or waveguides [3].

Now, the purpose of an electronic model of the brain is two-fold. First, it can be used to study the properties and function of the brain. Second, the model can be taken as the starting point in designing an electronic version of the brain, which can also help in designing human–machine interfaces and artificial intelligence systems.

There have been several attempts at representing biological neural networks by electronic networks. Starting with a single neuron, it can be simulated by a simple device with several inputs from other neurons and it acts as a threshold element which produces an output if the sum of the inputs exceeds a certain value. Then, a more elaborate definition allows the neuron to act as an exclusive OR gate, thus producing an output if and only if one input is nonzero. Thus it has an inhibitory action and is called a *perceptron*.

The learning function of neural networks is best simulated by the so-called electronic *artificial neural networks* (ANNs) and this approach allows the neurons to be interconnected in layers, as shown in figure 2.6. The processing takes place in the hidden layers whereas the input and output visible layers interface with the outside world and the learning or processing is achieved using interconnected nodes.

Thus an artificial neural network is an interconnected group of nodes, inspired by a simplified model of neurons in the brain. Here, each circular node represents an artificial neuron and an arrow represents a connection from the output of one artificial neuron to the input of another.

The circuit can be implemented in integrated circuit form and may be used to study the properties of biological neural networks and the brain functions and examine the effect of changing the various parameters. Of course, this idea can also be useful in designing intelligent machines or human–computer interfaces.

2.5 Accessing brain activity

Thus, the brain is an electronic signal processing system. To tap the electronic signal activities of the brain, there are several basic methods which include the following.

2.5.1 Electroencephalography (EEG)

A patient undergoing EEG is shown in figure 2.7, in which external electrodes are placed on the *scalp*. This yields somewhat indistinct outputs because the signals are attenuated and blurred by the scalp and skull.

2.5.2 Implants

Electrodes can be implanted *in the cortex*, as shown in figure 2.8. This gives clear results but requires surgery and penetration of the cortex. The implant causes scar tissue over time and carries the risks associated with invasive procedures.

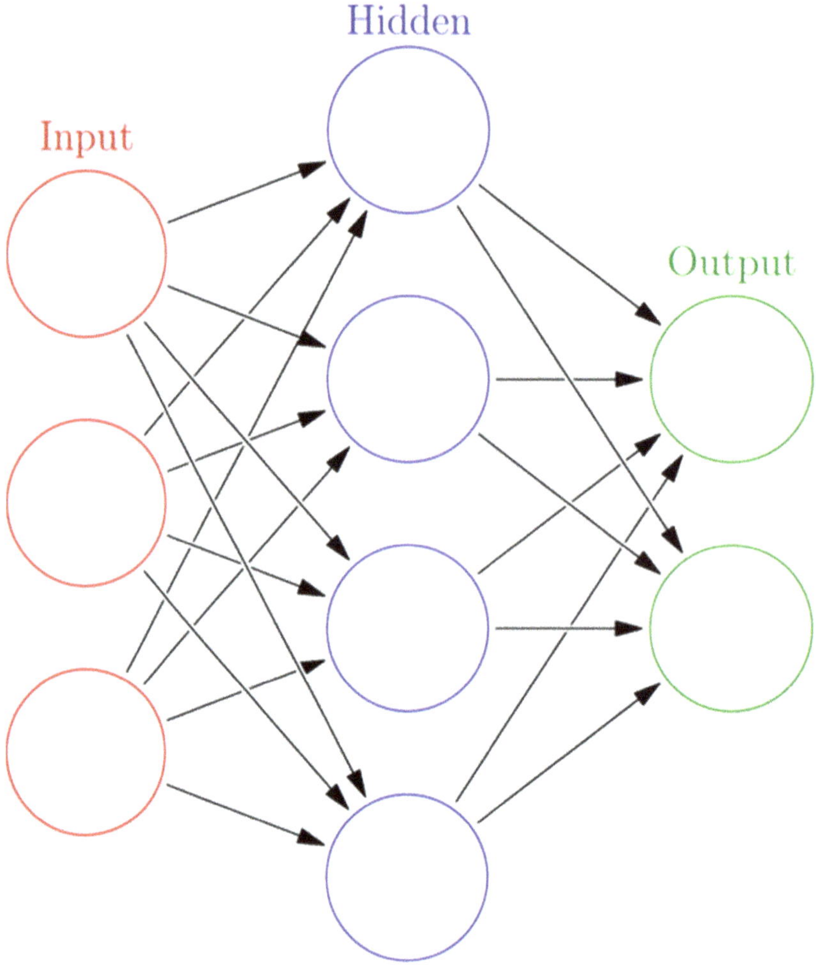

Figure 2.6. Machine learning with an Artificial Neural Network (ANN) [5]. *Source*: Glosser.ca https://commons.wikimedia.org/wiki/File:Colored_neural_network.svg CC BY-SA 3.0.

2.5.3 Electrocorticography (ECoG)

ECoG is shown in figure 2.9, in which electrodes are used in a *drape-like manner over the surface of the cortex*. This requires only penetration of the scull but not the cortex and therefore carries less risk than an implant while maintaining good clarity of brain activity and wider coverage by distributing the electrodes over a larger area.

2.6 Brain–machine interface and cortex mapping

Clearly, EEG, implants. or ECoG can be used to monitor and study brain activities. The EEG results for the alpha waves, which are the most prominent in a human EEG, occurring in the occipital lobe are shown in figure 2.10 and their spectrum lies in the frequency band between 7 and 13 Hz.

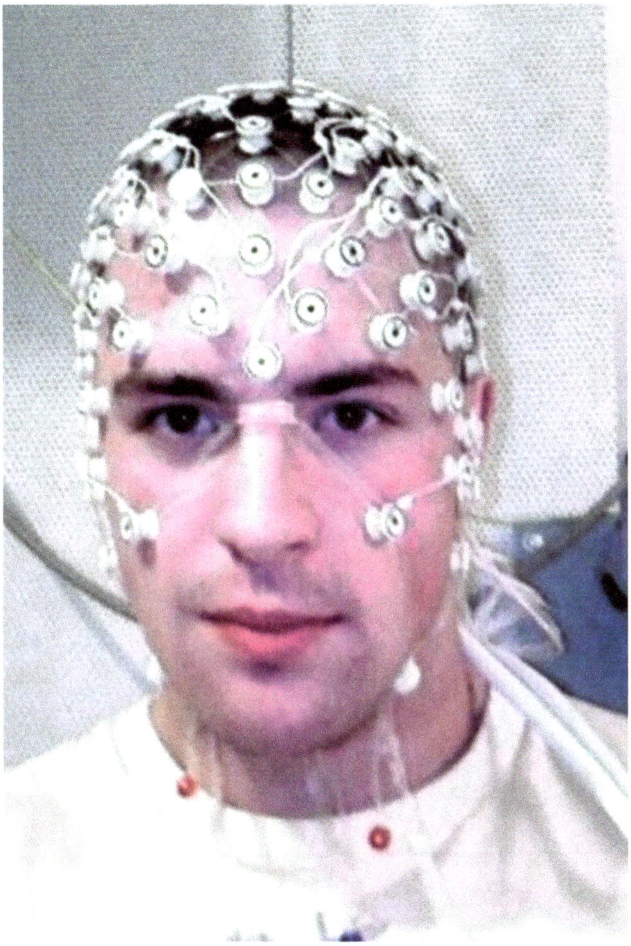

Figure 2.7. Electroencephalography (EEG) [6]. *Source*: thorThuglas https://commons.wikimedia.org/wiki/File:EEG_cap.jpg Public Domain.

These application can be extended far beyond mere monitoring. For example, the signals from certain parts of the cortex which appear at output are a result of thought processes, states of mind, and imagined movements. Recently it has been shown that alpha waves are modulated by the *intention* to act in a motor response. These can be fed into a computer system and converted into digital form then translated into movements of a robot arm or prosthesis or even speech. Thus, we have an example of a rudimentary brain–machine interface (BMI), as shown in figure 2.11.

In any event, both the electronic modelling of the brain and tapping the signals of its activity, form the bridge between electronic engineering and neuroscience. By placing the electrodes on the region of the brain associated with a certain activity like motor or sensory actions or speech, we can analyse the resulting signals and process them to replicate the activity.

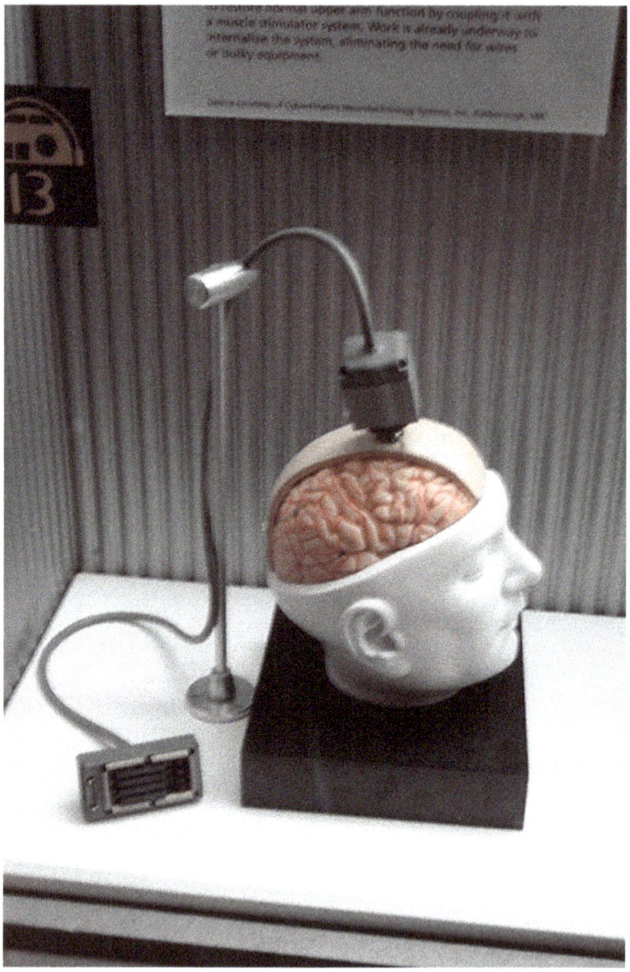

Figure 2.8. An implant [7]. *Source*: PaulWicks https://commons.wikimedia.org/wiki/File:BrainGate.jpg Public Domain.

Tapping brain signals also allows preparation for surgical procedures with assurance that the affected areas are the intended ones. By observing the signals, it is also possible to discover that certain frequency bands are associated with specific mental states. Moreover, certain frequency spectra correspond to specific movements. Therefore, a thorough spectral analysis of the output from the ECoG reveals a great deal about the brain. Some research groups have painstakingly and meticulously established the one-to-one correspondence between the positions of the electrodes spread over the cortex and certain signal spectra of the output of the ECoG.

The observation of brain signals has led to the establishment of fundamental properties of the sensorimotor parts, such as imagined movements and the discovery of mirror neurons and mu waves. A mirror neuron is one which is activated upon

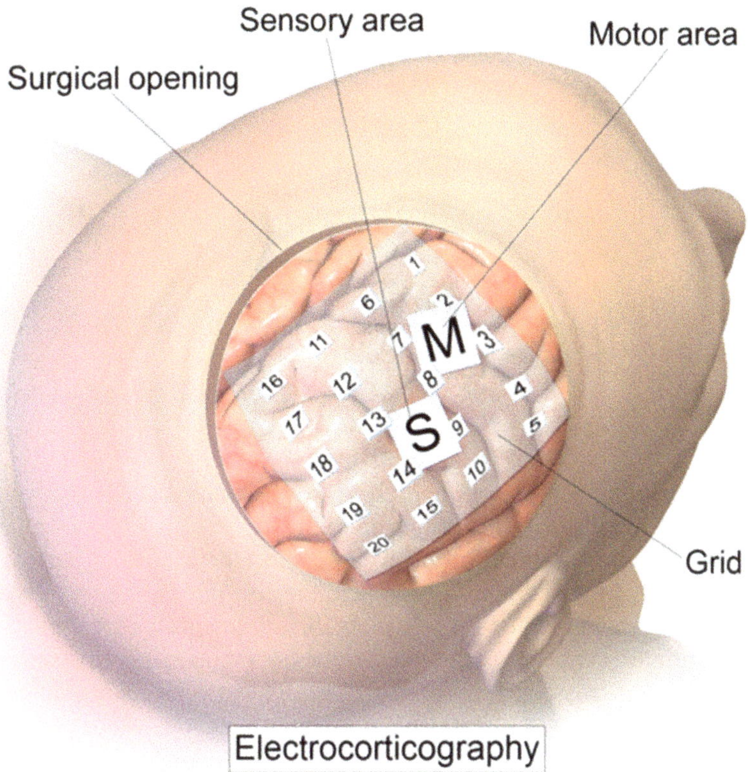

Figure 2.9. Electrocorticography (ECoG) [8]. *Source*: BruceBlaus https://commons.wikimedia.org/wiki/File:Intracranial_electrode_grid_for_electrocorticography.png CC BY-SA 3.0.

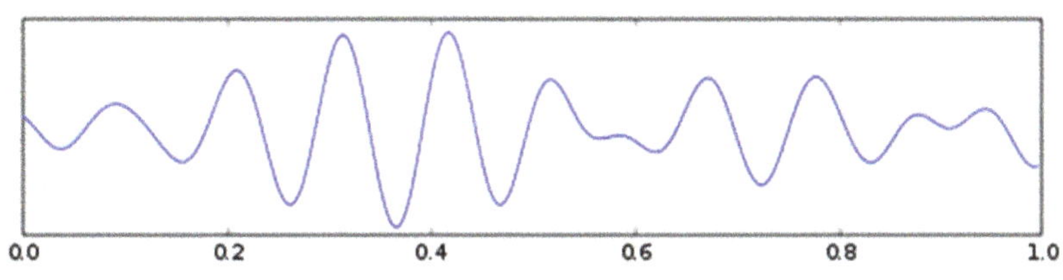

Figure 2.10. Alpha waves from EEG.

observation of an action performed by another person and the signal occupies a spectral band of 7–13 Hz. The mu waves occur in the motor cortex. Detection of modulated mu waves can be used to facilitate the movement of a paralysed person by simply *imagining* movement in order to trigger a response from a prothesis leading to *actual* external movement. This is similar to the scheme illustrated in figure 2.11.

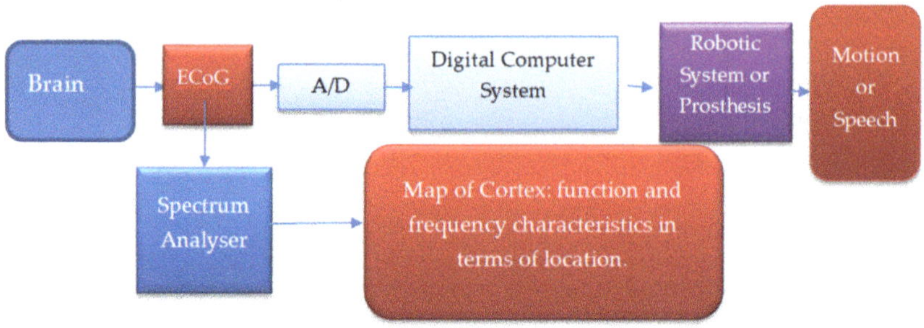

Figure 2.11. Using ECoG as part of a rudimentary brain–machine interface (BMI) and for the mapping of brain activities in terms of frequency response characteristics.

2.7 Conclusion

We have emphasised the nature of the brain as an electronic signal processing system and consequently the idea of modelling the brain and nervous system by electronic systems. These models continue to be developed and the road to a perfect model is necessarily infinitely long. The number of possible connections between the neurons in the brain is of the order of 10^{80}, which for all intents and purposes may be regarded as infinite. The electronic techniques for accessing the brain and its activities were also discussed, thus forming a bridge between electronic engineering and neuroscience.

References

[1] Baher H 1990 *Analog and Digital Signal Processing* (New York: Wiley)

[2] Baher H 2012 *Signal Processing and Integrated Circuits* (New York: Wiley)

[3] Baher H 1984 *Synthesis of Electrical Networks* (New York: Wiley)

[4] Kapooht 2013 File:Von Neumann Architecture.svg *Wikimedia Commons* https://commons.wikimedia.org/wiki/File:Von_Neumann_Architecture.svg

[5] Glosser.ca 2013 File:Colored neural network.svg *Wikimedia Commons* https://commons.wikimedia.org/wiki/File:Colored_neural_network.svg

[6] Thuglas 2010 File:EEG cap.jpg *Wikimedia Commons* https://commons.wikimedia.org/wiki/File:EEG_cap.jpg

[7] PaulWicks 2006 File:BrainGate.jpg *Wikimedia Commons* https://commons.wikimedia.org/wiki/File:BrainGate.jpg

[8] BruceBlaus 2014 File:Intracranial electrode grid for electrocorticography.png *Wikimedia Commons* https://commons.wikimedia.org/wiki/File:Intracranial_electrode_grid_for_electrocorticography.png

IOP Publishing

Electronic Engineering for Neuromedicine

Hussein Baher

Chapter 3

Neural signal processing

3.1 Introduction

One of the main topics of the hybrid field of *neural engineering* is the analysis and processing of neural signals. Signal processing includes two main areas: spectrum analysis and filtering. We have introduced spectrum analysis in the previous chapter. Here we discuss the filtering of signals in both the analog and digital domains and extend the spectrum analysis treatment to include power spectrum estimation of stochastic (random) signals, which is the real-life situation, in particular for neural signals.

3.2 Neural signals [1]

Throughout the previous chapters we have encountered several types of neural signals. These and others to be considered later in the book are summarised below.

1. Trains of impulses or spikes representing extracellular action potentials of the neurons.
2. Access to the brain is carried out using electrodes. In the vicinity of the electrodes extracellular signals exist which are called local field potential signals.
3. Electroencephalography (EEG) signals which result from currents flowing during the synaptic excitation of the dendrites in the neurons.
4. Magnetoencephalography (MEG) external magnetic field signals outside the head induced by signals resulting from intracellular currents flowing through dendrites. These are discussed later in the book.
5. Electrocorticography (ECoG) signals which are EEG recordings from the surface of the neocortex. These are localised high spatial-resolution signals.
6. Later in the book we shall encounter fMRI (functional magnetic resonance imaging) signals which measure variation in local blood volume, cerebral blood flow, and oxygenation levels induced by the neural activation by electromagnetic fields.
7. Calcium imaging signals which measure dynamic calcium flux within neurons and neuronal tissues.

doi:10.1088/978-0-7503-3427-3ch3

3.3 Filters and systems with frequency selectivity [2–4]

Here we consider the idealised situation of a linear time-invariant system (figure 3.1). In this case the system obeys the principle of superposition (increasing the input will proportionately increase the output) and the properties of the components do not vary with time. The transfer function of the system is the ratio of the output to the input in the frequency domain, i.e. it is the ratio of the Fourier transform of the response to the Fourier transform of the excitation:

$$H(\mathrm{j}\omega) = \frac{G(\mathrm{j}\omega)}{F(\mathrm{j}\omega)}$$

$$= |H(\mathrm{j}\omega)| \exp\,(\mathrm{j}\psi(\omega)).$$

By shaping this transfer function, a system with selective frequency response can be designed. This is the definition of a filter.

Also, any system has an inherent filtering characteristic by nature and not by design, i.e. an inherent frequency response. This means that, for example, a biological system does not have a flat frequency response not discriminating between various frequencies, instead it favours the transmission of certain frequencies as compared with other frequencies. We express this by stating that any system has a *bandwidth* within which the frequencies are transmitted without much attenuation and outside this bandwidth the frequencies are significantly attenuated. For example, the bandwidth of the human ear is between 20 and 20 kHz. Outside this range the frequencies are not heard. Therefore, the discussion of this section applies to both designed systems and naturally occurring biological systems.

The idealised frequency responses of filters are illustrated in figure 3.2.

The attenuation (or loss) function of a filter described by $H(\mathrm{j}\omega)$ is defined as (figure 3.3)

$$\alpha(\omega) = 10 \log \frac{1}{|H(\mathrm{j}\omega)|^2} \text{ dB}.$$

The ideal (no distortion) phase characteristic is a linear function of ω.

3.4 Digitisation of analog signals [5]

A signal $f(t)$ is called a *continuous-time* or an *analog* signal if it is defined, somehow, for all values of the *continuous* variable t. If $f(t)$ is defined only at discrete values of t,

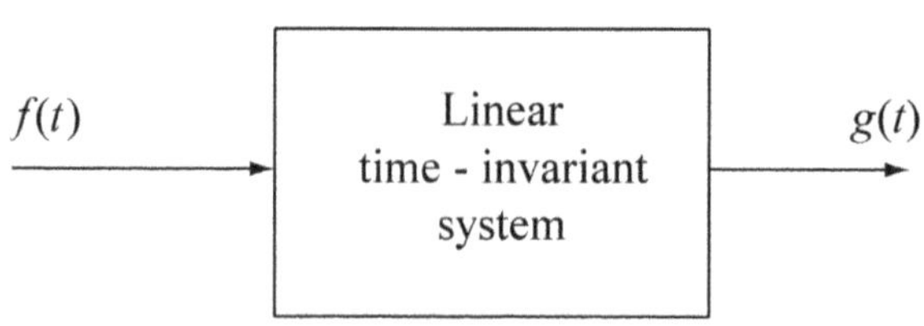

Figure 3.1. A linear system with input $f(t)$ and output $g(t)$.

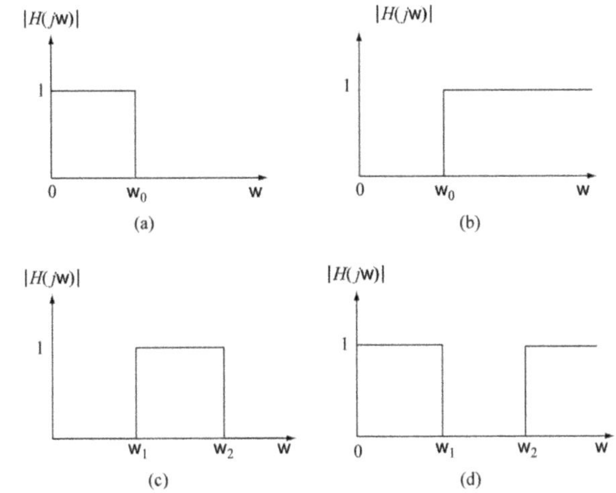

Figure 3.2. The ideal filter amplitude characteristics: (a) low-pass, (b) high-pass, (c) band-pass, and (d) band-stop.

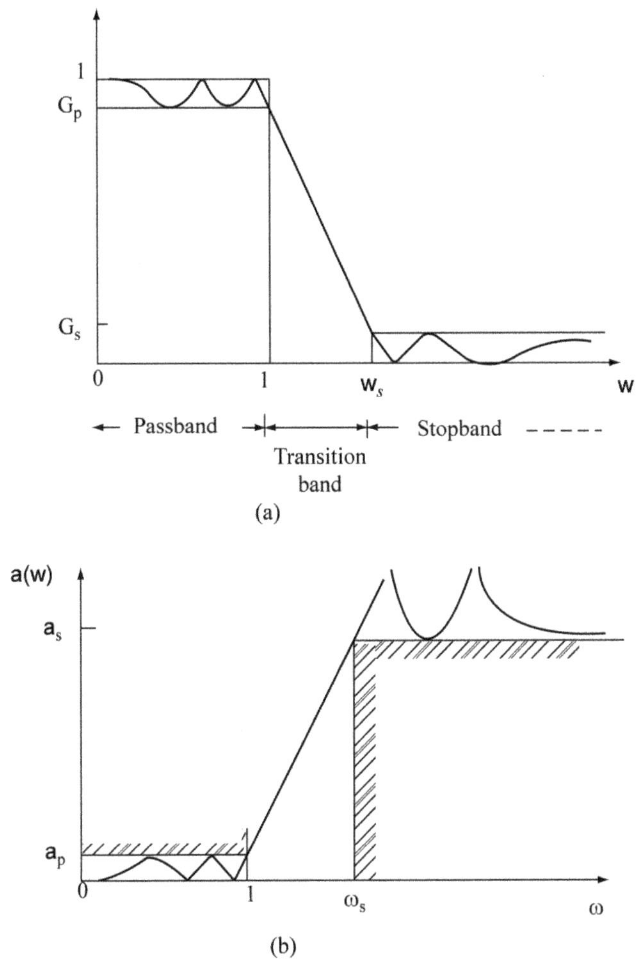

Figure 3.3. Tolerance scheme of a low-pass filter: (a) amplitude and (b) attenuation.

it is called a *discrete-time* signal or an *analog sampled-data* signal. Suppose that in addition to being discrete-time the signal quantities $f(t)$ can assume only discrete values, and that each value is represented by a code such as the binary code. The resulting signal is said to be a *digital signal.*

The first step in the digitisation process is to take samples of the signal $f(t)$ at regular time intervals: nT ($n = 0, \pm 1, \pm 2, \ldots$). This amounts to converting the continuous-time variable t into a discrete one. In this way we obtain a signal $f(nT)$ which is defined only at discrete instants which are integral multiples of the same quantity T, which is called the *sampling period.* Such a signal may be thought of as a sequence of numbers:

$$\{f(nT)\} \triangleq \{f(0),\ f(\pm T),\ f(\pm 2T),\ \ldots\}$$

representing the values of the function at the sampling instants. If the signal $f(t)$ is causal, i.e.

$$f(t) = 0 t < 0,$$

then the sampled version is denoted by the sequence

$$\{f(nT)\} \triangleq \{f(0),\ f(T),\ f(2T),\ \ldots\}.$$

Figure 3.4 shows a causal signal and its sampled version.

Next, the discrete-time signal is *quantised.* That is, the amplitude (vertical) axis is converted into a discrete one as shown in figure 3.4, and we regard the range of values between successive levels as inadmissible. Then, from the sequence $\{f(nT)\}$, we form a new *quantised* sequence $\{f_q(nT)\}$ by assigning to each $f(nT)$ the value of a quantisation level as shown in figure 3.5. Finally, the discrete-time quantised sequence $\{f_q(nT)\}$ is *encoded* as shown in figure 3.6. This means that each member of the sequence $\{f_q(nT)\}$ is represented by a code; the most commonly used one is a *binary* code.

The entire process of sampling, quantisation, and encoding is usually called *analog-to-digital (A/D) conversion.*

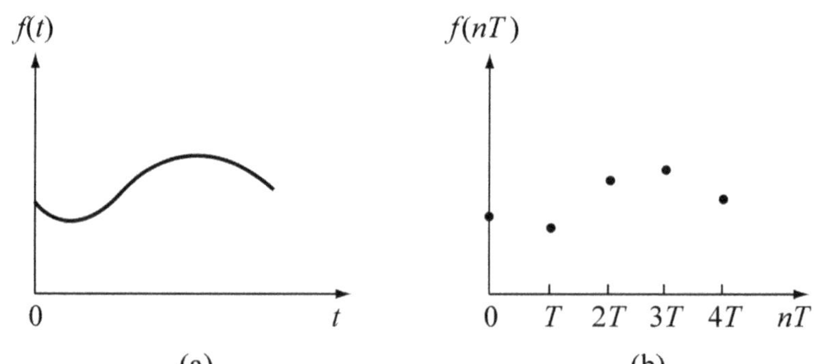

Figure 3.4. (a) A causal analog signal and (b) its sampled version.

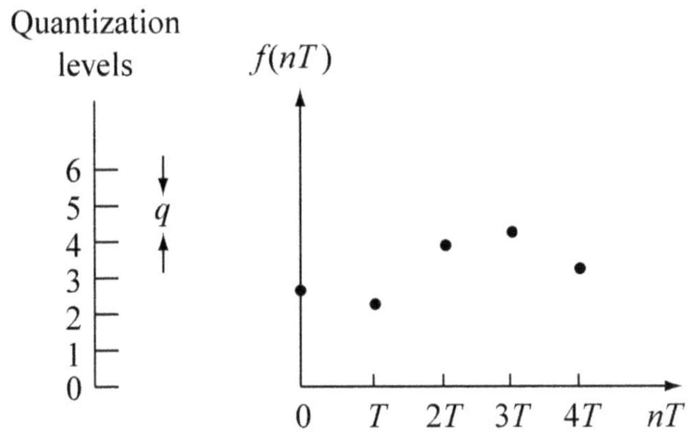

Figure 3.5. The sampled signal of figure 3.4 and the quantisation levels.

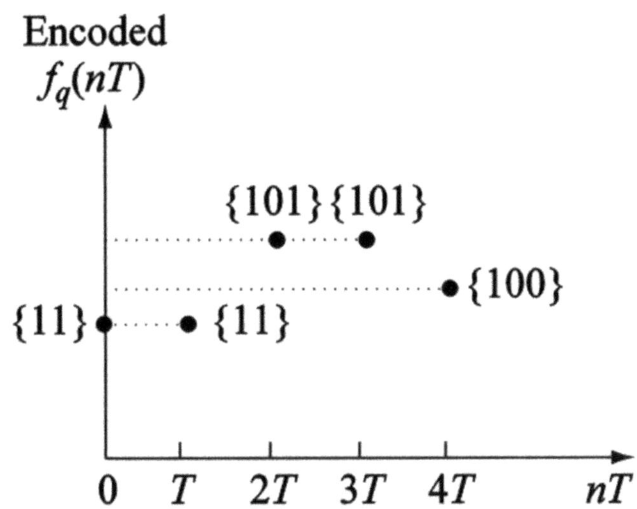

Figure 3.6. The digitised analog signal of figure 3.4 after quantisation and encoding.

In dealing with discrete signals, we use the *z-transformation* to have a frequency-domain representation analogous to that which we explained in the analog continuous-time domain. This is defined as

$$F(z) = Z\{f(n)\}$$

$$\stackrel{\Delta}{=} \sum_{n=0}^{\infty} f(n)z^{-n},$$

and the frequency-domain representation is obtained by letting

$$z^{-1} \equiv \exp(-\mathrm{j}T\omega).$$

3.5 Digital filters [3, 4]

A digital filter or system is described by a difference equation relating the input and the output as

$$g(n) = \sum_{r=0}^{M} a_r f(n-r) - \sum_{r=1}^{N} b_r g(n-r) \text{ with } M \leqslant N,$$

which is basically a recursion formula relating the input to the output sequences. In the z domain this leads to

$$G(z) = F(z)\sum_{r=0}^{M} a_r z^{-r} - G(z)\sum_{r=1}^{N} b_r z^{-r}$$

$$H(z) = \frac{G(z)}{F(z)}$$

$$H(z) = \frac{\sum_{r=0}^{M} a_r z^{-r}}{1 + \sum_{r=1}^{N} b_r z^{-r}}.$$

The building blocks of digital fitters are the multiplier, adder, and unit delay as shown in figure 3.7. These building blocks implement the transfer function of the filter using either software or hardware. They use logic gates which are simple transistor circuits realising logic functions such as AND, OR, and NOT operations.

A digital filter can be realised in the generic direct form as shown in figures 3.8 and 3.9.

3.6 Stochastic (random) signals [3–5]

Most signals are random, or at best contain random components. This is particularly true of neural signals and neuronal data. They are also weak signals which are susceptible to additive noise which introduces random components. Such signals require the use of statistical methods for their description. Neural signals and neuronal data cannot be treated exclusively using deterministic methods but because they often contain non-Gaussian non-stationary components, statistical and stochastic methods are required. For medical practitioners, the results of diagnostic tools are best understood if the analysis of these signals is given the correct interpretation. These considerations lead to the area of stochastic signal processing [3, 5]. *Throughout this chapter random quantities are denoted by boldface characters.*

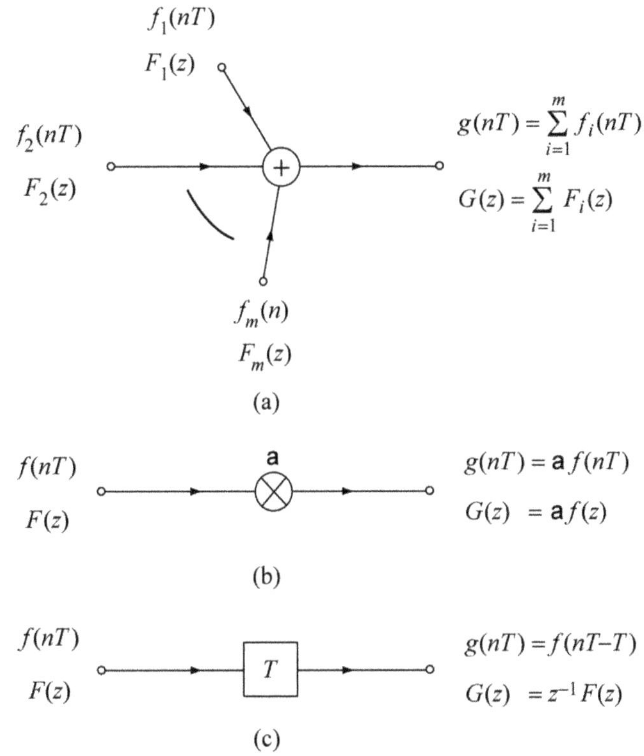

Figure 3.7. The basic building blocks of digital filters.

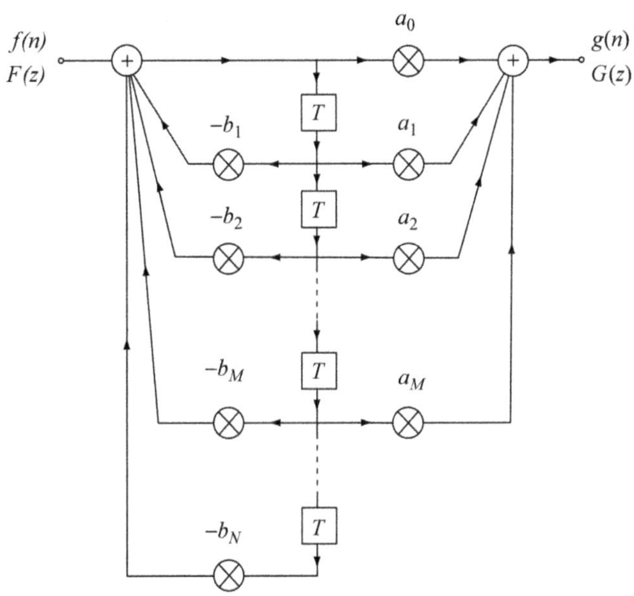

Figure 3.8. Direct realisation of a digital filter.

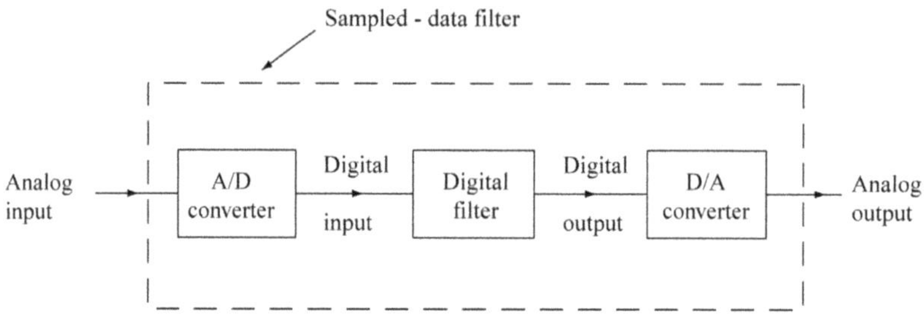

Figure 3.9. The digital filter in an analog environment.

3.6.1 Probability distribution function

Consider a random variable **f** which may take real values in a range $[f_1, f_2]$ where f_1 could be as low as $-\infty$ and f_2 as high as $+\infty$. Let us observe this variable over the entire range $[f_1, f_2]$ and define its *probability distribution function* as

$$P(f) \triangleq \text{Prob}[\mathbf{f} < f],$$

which is the probability that the random variable **f** assumes a value less than some given number f and we define the probability density function as

$$p(f) = \frac{\mathrm{d}P(f)}{\mathrm{d}f}.$$

This has the obvious property that

$$\int_{-\infty}^{\infty} p(f)\mathrm{d}f = 1$$

because any value of **f** must lie in the range $[-\infty, \infty]$. Moreover, the probability that **f** lies between f_1 and f_2 is given by

$$\text{Prob}\left[f_1 < \mathbf{f} < f_2\right] = \int_{f_1}^{f_2} p(f)\mathrm{d}f.$$

The shape of the probability density function curve indicates the 'preferred' range of values which **f** assumes. For example, a commonly occurring probability density function is the Gaussian one given by

$$p(f) = \frac{1}{(2\pi\sigma)^{1/2}} \exp[-(f - \eta)^2/2\sigma^2],$$

where σ and η are constants. This is shown in figure 3.10. Another example is the case shown in figure 3.11 where there is no preferred range for the random variable **f** between f_1 and f_2. The probability density is said to be *uniform* and is given by

$$\begin{aligned} p(f) &= 1/(f_2 - f_1) \qquad f_1 \leqslant \mathbf{f} \leqslant f_2 \\ &= 0 \qquad \text{otherwise.} \end{aligned}$$

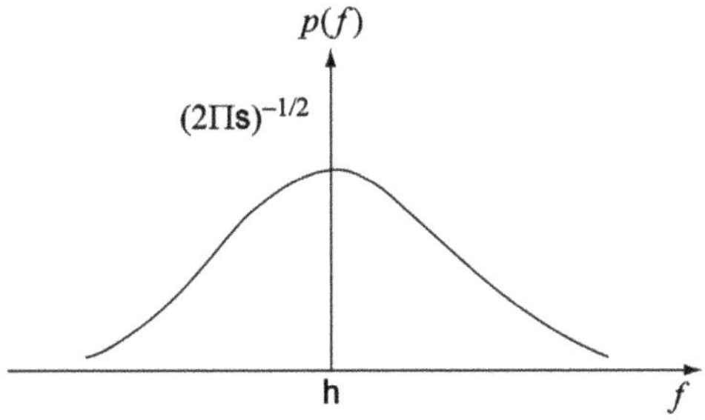

Figure 3.10. Gaussian probability density function defined.

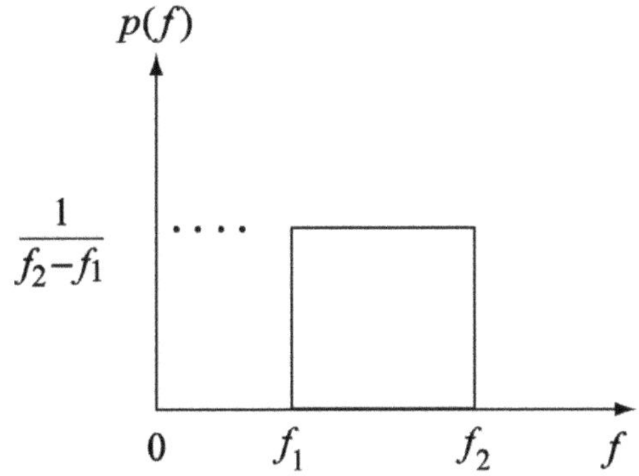

Figure 3.11. Uniform probability density function.

The probability of observing **f** and **g** below f and g, respectively, is referred to as the *joint distribution function* of **f** and **g**:

$$P(f, g) = \text{Prob}[\mathbf{f} < f, \mathbf{g} < g].$$

The *joint probability density function* of **f** and **g** is defined by

$$p(f, g) = \frac{\partial^2 P(f, g)}{\partial f \, \partial g}.$$

Again, since the range $[-\infty, \infty]$ includes **f** and **g** we must have

$$\int_{-\infty}^{\infty}\int_{-\infty}^{\infty} p(f, g)\mathrm{d}f\,\mathrm{d}g = 1.$$

The two random variables **f** and **g** representing the outcomes (ζ_{f1}, ζ_{f2}, …) and (ζ_{g1}, ζ_{g2}, …) are said to be *statistically independent* if the occurrence of any outcome ζ_g does not affect the occurrence of any outcome ζ_f and vice versa. This is the case if and only if

$$p(f, g) = p(f)p(g).$$

The description of the properties of random variables can be accomplished by means of a number of parameters. These are now reviewed.

(i) *The mean or first moment, or expectation value* of a random variable **f** is denoted by $E[\mathbf{f}]$ or η_f and is defined by

$$E[\mathbf{f}] \triangleq \int_{-\infty}^{\infty} f\, p(f)\mathrm{d}f$$

$$\equiv \eta_f .$$

More generally, if a random variable **u** is a function of two other random variables **f** and **g**, i.e.

$$\mathbf{u} \triangleq \mathbf{u}(\mathbf{f}, \mathbf{g}),$$

then

$$E[\mathbf{u}] = \int_{-\infty}^{\infty} u\, p(u)\mathrm{d}u$$

and

$$\mathrm{Prob}[u < \mathbf{u} < u + \mathrm{d}u] = \mathrm{Prob}[f < \mathbf{f} < f + \mathrm{d}f,\ g < \mathbf{g} < g + \mathrm{d}g],$$

i.e.

$$p(u)\mathrm{d}u = p(f,\ g)\mathrm{d}f\,\mathrm{d}g,$$

which, upon use of (4.14), gives

$$E[\mathbf{u}] = \int_{-\infty}^{\infty}\int_{-\infty}^{\infty} u(f,\ g)p(f, g)\mathrm{d}f\,\mathrm{d}g.$$

In the special case of

$$\mathbf{u} = \mathbf{fg}$$

we have

$$E[\mathbf{fg}] = \int_{-\infty}^{\infty}\int_{-\infty}^{\infty} f\,g\,p(f,\ g)\ \mathrm{d}f\,\mathrm{d}g.$$

Furthermore, if **f** and **g** are independent variables, then

$$E[\mathbf{fg}] = \int_{-\infty}^{\infty} f\,p(f)\mathrm{d}f \int_{-\infty}^{\infty} g\,p(g)\mathrm{d}g$$

$$= E[\mathbf{f}]E[\mathbf{g}].$$

It is always possible to 'centre' the variable by subtracting from it, its mean η; this gives the centred variable $\mathbf{f}_c$ as

$$\mathbf{f}_c = \mathbf{f} - \eta$$

$$= \mathbf{f} - E[\mathbf{f}],$$

which is a *zero-mean* variable.

The second central moment of **f** is given by

$$E[\mathbf{f}_c^2] = E[(\mathbf{f} - \eta)^2].$$

Noting that the expectation operator $E[\cdot]$ is linear, we have

$$E[(\mathbf{f} - \eta)^2] = E[\mathbf{f}^2] - E[2\eta \mathbf{f}] + \eta^2$$

$$= E[\mathbf{f}^2] - 2\eta E[\mathbf{f}] + \eta^2$$

$$= E[\mathbf{f}^2] - \eta^2.$$

(ii) *The central second moment* is called the *variance* of **f** and is denoted by σ_f^2. Thus

$$\sigma_f^2 = E[\mathbf{f}^2] - \eta^2$$

$$= E[\mathbf{f}^2] - E^2[\mathbf{f}].$$

For a uniform distribution

$$E[\mathbf{f}] = \int_{f_1}^{f_2} \frac{f}{f_2 - f_1}\, \mathrm{d}f = \frac{1}{2}(f_1 + f_2)$$

$$= \eta$$

$$E[\mathbf{f}^2] = \int_{f_1}^{f_2} \frac{f^2}{f_2 - f_1}\, \mathrm{d}f = \frac{f_2^3 - f_1^3}{3(f_2 - f_1)}.$$

Substituting from the above two expressions into (4.24) we obtain for the variance

$$\sigma_f^2 = \frac{(f_2 - f_1)^2}{12}.$$

For a Gaussian distribution

$$E[\mathbf{f}] = \eta_f = \eta$$

and

$$E[\mathbf{f}^2] = \sigma^2 + \eta^2$$

or

$$\sigma_f^2 = \sigma^2.$$

We denote the stochastic process by $\mathbf{f}(t, \zeta)$, and for simplicity we often drop the parameter ζ and denote the process by $\mathbf{f}(t)$.

From the above definitions we see that a stochastic process is an infinite number of random variables—one for every t (figure 3.12). For a specific t, $\mathbf{f}(t)$ is, therefore, a random variable with probability distribution function

$$P(f, t) = \mathrm{Prob}[\mathbf{f}(t) < f],$$

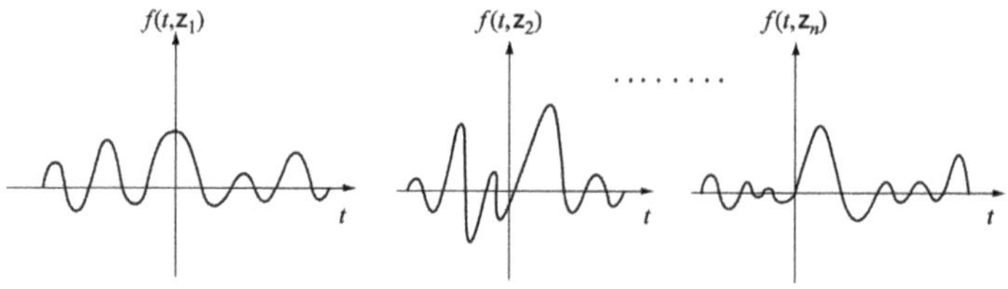

Figure 3.12. Analog stochastic process as an ensemble of samples.

which depends on t, and it is equal to the probability of the *event* ($\mathbf{f}(t) < f$) consisting of all outcomes ζ_i such that at the specific time t, the samples $\mathbf{f}(t, \zeta_i)$ of the given process are below the number f. The partial derivative of $P(f, t)$ with respect to f is the probability density

$$p(f, t) = \frac{\partial P(f, t)}{\partial f}.$$

In which $P(f, t)$ is called the first-order distribution, and $p(f, t)$ is the first-order density of the process $\mathbf{f}(t)$.

At two specific instants t_1 and t_2, $\mathbf{f}(t_1)$ and $\mathbf{f}(t_2)$ are distinct random variables. Their joint probability distribution is given by

$$P(f_1, f_2;\, t_1, t_2) = \text{Prob}\left[\mathbf{f}(t_1) < f_1;\, \mathbf{f}(t_2) < f_2\right]$$

and their probability density function is

$$p(f_1, f_2;\, t_1, t_2) = \frac{\partial^2 P(f_1, f_2;\, t_1, t_2)}{\partial f_1\, \partial f_2}.$$

In order to possess complete information about the properties of a stochastic process, we must know the probability distribution function $P[f_1, f_2, \ldots, f_n; t_1, t_2, \ldots, t_n]$ for every f_i, t_i, and n. For many applications only the expected values $E[\mathbf{f}(t)]$ and $E[\mathbf{f}^2(t)]$ are used to characterise the process. These are the second-order properties of the process. For any t, *the mean* $\eta(t)$ of $\mathbf{f}(t)$ is the expected value of the random variable $\mathbf{f}(t)$,

$$\eta(t) = E[\mathbf{f}(t)] = \int_{-\infty}^{\infty} f\, p(f, t)\mathrm{d}f.$$

The *mean square* of the process is given by

$$E[\mathbf{f}^2(t)] = \int_{-\infty}^{\infty} f^2 p(f, t)\mathrm{d}f.$$

The *autocorrelation* $R_{ff}(t_1, t_2)$ is defined as the expected value (or mean) of the product $\mathbf{f}(t_1)\mathbf{f}(t_2)$, thus

$$R_{ff}(t_1, t_2) = E[\mathbf{f}(t_1)\mathbf{f}(t_2)]$$

$$= \int_{-\infty}^{\infty}\int_{-\infty}^{\infty} P(f_1, f_2;\, t_1, t_2)\mathrm{d}f_1\,\mathrm{d}f_2$$

$$= R_{ff}(t_2, t_1).$$

This parameter is a measure of the inter-relatedness between the instantaneous signal values at t_1 and those at t_2. For $t_1 = t_2 = t$,

$$R_{ff}(t, t) = E[\mathbf{f}^2(t)] \geqslant 0,$$

which is the mean square of the process and is called the *average power* of $\mathbf{f}(t)$. In fact the autocorrelation is the single most important property of a random process since it leads to a frequency-domain representation of the process.

The *cross-correlation* of two processes $\mathbf{f}(t)$ and $\mathbf{g}(t)$ is denoted by $R_{fg}(t_1, t_2)$ and is defined as the expected value of the product $\mathbf{f}(t_1)\mathbf{g}(t_2)$; thus

$$R_{fg}(t_1, t_2) = E[\mathbf{f}(t_1)\mathbf{g}(t_2)].$$

The *cross-covariance* $C_{fg}(t_1, t_2)$ is defined as the expectation of the product

$$\left\{\mathbf{f}(t_1) - \eta_f(t_1)\right\}\left\{\mathbf{g}(t_2) - \eta_g(t_2)\right\},$$

where η_f and η_g are the means of $f(t)$ and $g(t)$, respectively. Thus

$$C_{fg}(t_1, t_2) = E\left[\left\{\mathbf{f}(t_1) - \eta_f(t_1)\right\}\left\{\mathbf{g}(t_2) - \eta_g(t_2)\right\}\right].$$

Using the linearity of the expectation operator,

$$C_{fg}(t_1, t_2) = E[\mathbf{f}(t_1)\mathbf{g}(t_2)] - \eta_f(t_1)\eta_g(t_2),$$

which, upon use of (7.40), becomes

$$C_{fg}(t_1, t_2) = R_{fg}(t_1, t_2) - \eta_f(t_1)\eta_g(t_2).$$

The *auto-covariance* of a random process $\mathbf{f}(t)$ is denoted by $C_{ff}(t_1, t_2)$ and is obtained as

$$C_{ff}(t) = R_{ff}(t, t) - \eta_f^2,$$

which is the *variance* of $\mathbf{f}(t)$.

3.6.2 Stationary processes

A stochastic process is said to be *strictly stationary* if all its statistical properties are invariant to a shift of the time origin, i.e. all its properties are independent of time. On the other hand, the process is called *wide-sense stationary* if its mean is independent of time, and its autocorrelation depends only on the difference $\tau = t_1 - t_2$.

3.7 Power spectra of stochastic signals

We have seen that for a deterministic finite-energy signal $f(t)$, the autocorrelation function $\rho_{ff}(\tau)$ and its energy spectrum $E(\omega)$ constitute a Fourier transform pair, as expressed by the relation

$$\rho_{ff}(\tau) \leftrightarrow E(\omega),$$

where

$$E(\omega) = F(\omega)F^*(\omega)$$
$$= |F(\omega)|^2,$$

with

$$f(t) \leftrightarrow F(\omega),$$

i.e.

$$\rho_{ff}(\tau) \leftrightarrow \left|F(\omega)\right|^2.$$

Moreover, the cross-correlation $\rho_{fg}(\tau)$ of two finite-energy signals $f(t)$ and $g(t)$, together with the cross-energy spectrum $F^*(\omega)G(\omega) = E_{fg}(\omega)$ form a Fourier transform pair, i.e.

$$\rho_{fg}(\tau) \leftrightarrow F^*(\omega)G(\omega).$$

Turning now to stochastic signals, we note that these are not square integrable and, in general, do not possess Fourier transforms. Therefore, we seek an alternative frequency-domain representation of the statistical properties of such signals. This is usually accomplished in terms of their *power spectra*, rather than the energy spectra. We shall concentrate on stationary signals which are also mean-ergodic and correlation-ergodic.

The power spectral density, or simply the *power spectrum* $P_{ff}(\omega)$ of a stationary process $\mathbf{f}(t)$, is defined as the Fourier transform of its autocorrelation, i.e.

$$P_{ff}(\omega) = \int_{-\infty}^{\infty} R_{ff}(\tau)\exp(-\mathrm{j}\omega\, t)\mathrm{d}\tau$$

with the inverse relation

$$R_{ff}(\tau) = \frac{1}{2\pi}\int_{-\infty}^{\infty} P_{ff}(\omega)\exp(\mathrm{j}\omega\,\tau)\mathrm{d}\omega$$

so that we have the Fourier transform pair

$$R_{ff}(\tau) \leftrightarrow P_{ff}(\omega)$$

zero frequency.

For a correlation-ergodic process, the autocorrelation, hence the power spectrum, can be obtained from time averages as

$$R_{ff}(\tau) = \lim_{T\to\infty}\frac{1}{T}\int_{-T/2}^{T/2} \mathbf{f}(t)\mathbf{f}(t+\tau)\mathrm{d}t.$$

This forms the basis for the estimation of the power spectrum of a stochastic process. The process is observed over a sufficiently large period and the expression

$$R_{ff}(\tau) \approx \frac{1}{T}\int_{-T/2}^{T/2} \mathbf{f}(t)\mathbf{f}(t+\tau)\mathrm{d}t$$

is taken as an estimate of the autocorrelation.

3.7.1 Cross-power spectrum

For two jointly stationary processes $\mathbf{f}(t)$ and $\mathbf{g}(t)$, the cross-power spectrum $P_{fg}(\omega)$ is defined as the Fourier transform of their cross-correlation. Thus

$$P_{fg}(\omega) = \int_{-\infty}^{\infty} R_{fg}(\tau)\exp(-\mathrm{j}\omega\,\tau)\mathrm{d}\tau$$

with the inverse relation

$$R_{fg}(\tau) = \frac{1}{2\pi}\int_{-\infty}^{\infty} P_{fg}(\omega)\exp(\mathrm{j}\omega\,\tau)\mathrm{d}\omega$$

so that the cross-correlation and the cross-power spectrum (density) form a Fourier transform pair

$$R_{fg}(\tau) \leftrightarrow P_{fg}(\omega).$$

Again, for correlation-ergodic jointly stationary processes, the cross-correlation can be obtained from the time average

$$R_{fg}(\tau) = \lim_{T\to\infty}\frac{1}{T}\int_{-T/2}^{T/2} \mathbf{f}(t)\mathbf{g}(t+\tau)\mathrm{d}t,$$

which is equal to the ensemble average. The cross-power spectrum has the property

$$P_{fg}(\omega) = P^{*}_{fg}(\omega).$$

We obtain for stationary correlation-ergodic processes

$$P_{fg}(\omega) = P^{*}_{ff}(\omega)P_{gg}(\omega).$$

3.7.2 White noise

A random process whose power spectrum is constant at all frequencies is called *white noise*. For such a signal

$$P_{\mathrm{WN}}(\omega) = A \text{ (a constant)},$$

so that its inverse Fourier transform gives its autocorrelation as

$$R_{\mathrm{WN}}(\tau) = A\delta(\tau),$$

which is an impulse at $\tau = 0$.

Figure 3.13 shows some autocorrelation functions and the corresponding power spectra. Figure 3.13(a) is white noise and figure 3.13(b) is a band-limited white noise. Figure 3.13(c) represents thermal noise through a resistor.

3.8 Power spectrum estimation [3, 5]

A problem of considerable importance in signal processing is that of the *estimation* of the power spectrum $P_{ff}(\omega)$ of a process $\mathbf{f}(t)$ when only a segment $\mathbf{f}_T(t)$ is available. If the autocorrelation $R_{ff}(\tau)$ is *known* for every τ in the interval $[-T/2, T/2]$ then fast

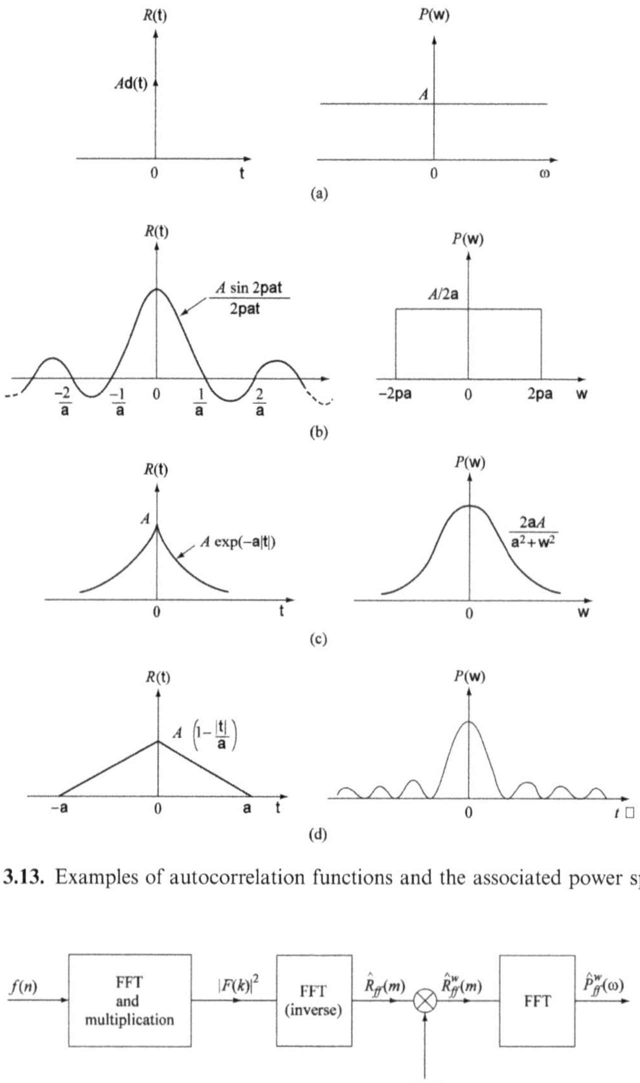

Figure 3.13. Examples of autocorrelation functions and the associated power spectra.

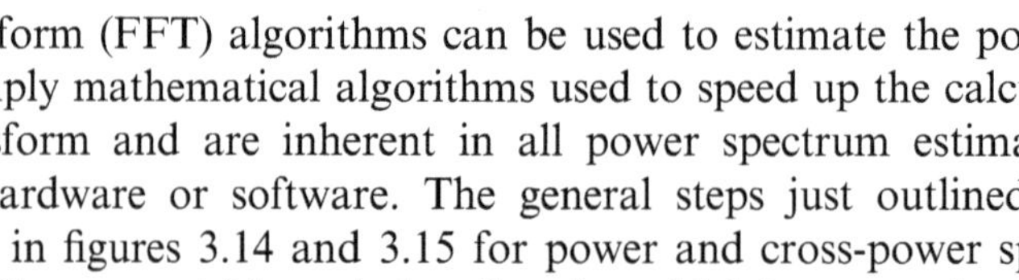

Figure 3.14. Power spectrum estimation using FFT algorithms.

Fourier transform (FFT) algorithms can be used to estimate the power spectrum. These are simply mathematical algorithms used to speed up the calculations of the Fourier transform and are inherent in all power spectrum estimation methods whether in hardware or software. The general steps just outlined are depicted schematically in figures 3.14 and 3.15 for power and cross-power spectra, respectively. In the diagrams $w(n)$ is a window function which improves the accuracy of the calculations by reducing the inherent errors. All the operations are carried out using special software which is built in the spectrum analysers used for the power spectrum estimation. Here we speak of estimation rather that determination because we are

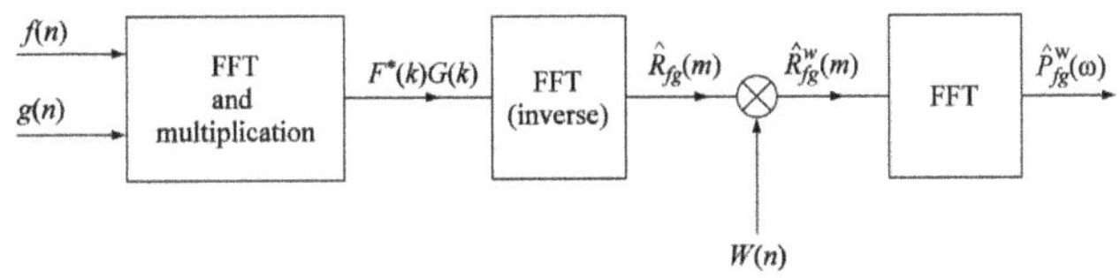

Figure 3.15. Cross-power spectrum estimation using FFT algorithms.

dealing with stochastic (random) signals whose properties can only be evaluated using probabilistic and statistical methods.

3.9 Conclusion

Accessing brain signals, as discussed in chapter 2, is the preparatory phase of neural signal processing. The next step involves spectrum analysis and filtering. Since the neural signals and neuronal data are noisy and inherently stochastic, this chapter discussed filtering in both the analog and digital domains as well as power spectrum estimation of stochastic signals and the statistical parameters used to characterize such signals. These topics are necessary for the correct interpretation and understanding of the accessed neuronal data and neural signals.

References

[1] Chen Z 2017 A primer on neural signal processing *IEEE Circuits Syst. Mag.* **17** 33–50 March
[2] Baher H 1984 *Synthesis of Electrical Networks* (New York: Wiley)
[3] Baher H 2012 *Signal Processing and Integrated Circuits* (New York: Wiley)
[4] Baher H 1996 *Microelectronic Switched Capacitor Filters* (New York: Wiley)
[5] Baher H 1990 *Analog and Digital Signal Processing* (New York: Wiley)

IOP Publishing

Electronic Engineering for Neuromedicine

Hussein Baher

Chapter 4

Electronic psychiatry

4.1 Introduction

There was a time when a patient would ask a psychiatrist whether he was a *talking* psychiatrist or a *drug* psychiatrist. The time has come when a third option is available, namely that of an *electronic* psychiatrist! Since the realisation that the nervous system is fundamentally an electronic system as well as an electro-chemical one, attempts have been made to influence the behaviour of the system from outside using electric and magnetic means in a manner that minimises the use of drugs or surgery, or eliminates them altogether. The earliest type of such therapy was the electroconvulsive treatment, which has been used in cases which do not respond to drugs but has had the notoriety of causing amnesia and has always been dreaded by patients, with close associations with the Frankenstein story and the film *One Flew over the Cuckoo's Nest* in which it was used as a punishment.

Alternatives are now available [1–7]. These rely on the use of electromagnetic fields to design devices for the triggering of favourable responses from neurons. The aim is to counteract the psychopathological conditions of patients. These have been used for the treatment of ailments such as epilepsy, depression, and obsessive compulsive disorder (OCD) using electric pulses or electromagnets.

Furthermore, the digital revolution and the wide-spread use of smart phones and wearable devices have opened a new horizon which may be called *digital psychiatry*. The combination of smart devices and tracking applications incorporating sensors, GPS, Bluetooth, near field communication (NFC), accelerometers, and gyroscopes are being used for the diagnosis, monitoring, and treatment of psychological disorders.

4.2 Magnetic fields and electromagnetic field theory

In chapter 1 we gave a summary of electric field theory. In this section we complete the picture by giving a brief summary of magnetic fields and combine the results of chapter 1 to form *electromagnetic field theory* which will facilitate the comprehension of the subsequent applications. This is currently important since the basic education of many

doi:10.1088/978-0-7503-3427-3ch4

science and medical students lacks the rigorous treatment of electromagnetic fields. Sadly, this created a gap in the intellectual makeup of science, engineering, and medical professionals causing difficulties and problems (yes! not 'challenges' and 'issues', the fashionable meaningless terms used nowadays). Science *solves problems* and *overcomes difficulties*; it does not 'address issues' and 'meet challenges'. The next section is an attempt to fill this gap with the absolute minimum of detail.

4.2.1 The Biot–Savart law (Laplace's rule)

The basic unit source of magnetic field is the current-carrying conductor (figure 4.1). The magnetic field intensity $\mathrm{d}\vec{H}$ at any point P, produced by a current-carrying element is

$$\mathrm{d}\vec{H} = \frac{I\mathrm{d}\vec{\ell} \times \vec{a}_r}{4\pi r^2}\ \mathrm{A\ m^{-1}},$$

where

$\mathrm{d}\vec{\ell}$ = vector element pointing in the direction of I.

$\vec{a}_r$ = unit vector from $d\vec{\ell}$ to P.

r = distance from $d\vec{\ell}$ to P.

Thus $\mathrm{d}\vec{H}$ is normal to the plane formed by the current-carrying element $\mathrm{d}\vec{\ell}$ and the vector $\vec{r}$.

Then for a current-carrying conductor

$$\vec{H} = \oint_C \frac{I\mathrm{d}\vec{\ell} \times \vec{a}_r}{4\pi r^2}\ \mathrm{A\ m^{-1}}.$$

The cross or vector product in the integral is defined as a vector of magnitude equalling the product of the two magnitudes times the sine of the angle between the two and has a direction normal to the plane formed by the two vectors.

4.2.2 Ampere's circuital law

The line integral of the tangential component of $\vec{H}$ around any closed path is the current enclosed by that path:

$$\oint_C \vec{H} \cdot \mathrm{d}\vec{\ell} = I.$$

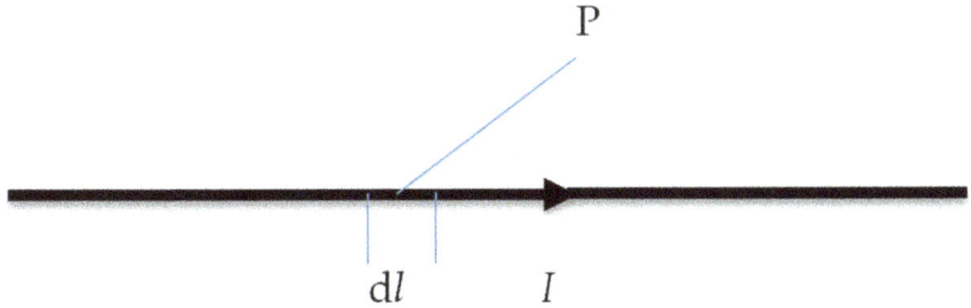

Figure 4.1. A current-carrying conductor.

Very often the magnetic field is generated using coils in the form of circular conductors wound with or without iron cores. The magnetic field at the centre of a circular loop of radius R carrying a current I is given by

$$H = \frac{I}{2\pi R}.$$

4.2.3 Stokes' theorem

Consider a closed path C, enclosing an open surface S. Then Stokes' theorem is given by

$$\oint_C \vec{H} \cdot \mathrm{d}\vec{\ell} = \int_S \left(\nabla \times \vec{H}\right) \cdot \mathrm{d}\vec{S},$$

where

$$\nabla \times \vec{H} = \mathrm{curl}\vec{H} = \begin{vmatrix} \vec{i} & \vec{j} & \vec{k} \\ \frac{\partial}{\partial x} & \frac{\partial}{\partial y} & \frac{\partial}{\partial z} \\ H_x & H_y & H_z \end{vmatrix}.$$

Stokes' theorem is general and applies to any vector, not just $\vec{H}$, so we may write in general for any vector $\vec{F}$:

$$\oint_C \vec{F} \cdot \mathrm{d}\vec{\ell} = \int_S \left(\nabla \times \vec{F}\right) \cdot \mathrm{d}\vec{S}.$$

Using Ampere's circuital law,

$$\oint_C \vec{H} \cdot \mathrm{d}\vec{\ell} = I = \int_S \vec{J} \cdot \mathrm{d}\vec{S},$$

in which J is the current density, i.e. the current per unit area. When combined with Stokes' theorem

$$\vec{J} = \mathrm{curl}\vec{H}.$$

4.2.4 The magnetic flux density

The way in which electric fields may be detected is through the force exerted on static charges placed in these fields. Similarly, magnetic fields can be detected by the forces acting on moving charges (note: single magnetic poles do not exist in nature: only dipoles do). These forces always depend on the medium.

The magnetic vector corresponding to the electric field intensity is called the magnetic flux density $\vec{B}$. In free space

$$\vec{B} = \mu_0 \vec{H}$$

$$\mu_0 = 4\pi \times 10^{-7}\ \mathrm{H\,m^{-1}}.$$

In general

$$\vec{B} = \mu\vec{H}$$

$$\mu = \mu_r\mu_0,$$

where
μ_r = relative permeability
μ_0 = permeability of free space.
The *magnetic flux* is

$$\varphi = \int_S \vec{B} \cdot d\vec{S}$$

the units are webers.

The lines of magnetic flux do not have either sources or sinks and are always closed on themselves since individual isolated magnetic 'poles' equivalent to point charges are not known to exist:

$$\therefore \oint_S \vec{B} \cdot d\vec{S} = 0.$$

4.2.5 Gauss' theorem

$$\int (\text{div}\,\vec{B})dv = 0$$

$$\text{div}\vec{B} = 0$$

$$\nabla \cdot \vec{B} = 0.$$

The inductance describes the effect of magnetic energy storage in an electric circuit:

$$L = \frac{1}{I}\int_S \vec{B} \cdot d\vec{S} = \frac{\varphi}{I}.$$

The relation between the electromotive force (e.m.f.) induced in a closed loop and the magnetic field producing this e.m.f. is given by the empirical result known as Faraday's law of electromagnetic induction:

The e.m.f. induced in any closed path is equal to the time rate of change of the magnetic flux linking that path. The induced e.m.f. is always in such a direction as to produce a current whose flux opposes the change in the flux:

$$\text{e. m. f.} = -\frac{d\varphi}{dt}$$

$$\oint \vec{E}_i \cdot \mathrm{d}\vec{l} = -\frac{\partial \varphi}{\partial t}$$

$$= -\frac{\partial}{\partial t} \oint_S \vec{B} \cdot \mathrm{d}\vec{S}$$

$$= -\oint_S \frac{\partial \vec{B}}{\partial t} \cdot \mathrm{d}\vec{S}.$$

But from Stokes' theorem,

$$\oint_C \vec{E} \cdot \mathrm{d}\vec{l} = \int_S \left(\nabla \times \vec{E}\right) \cdot \mathrm{d}\vec{S}$$

$$= -\int_S \frac{\partial \vec{B}}{\partial t} \cdot \mathrm{d}\vec{S}$$

$$\nabla \times \vec{E} = -\frac{\partial \vec{B}}{\partial t}$$

or

$$\nabla \times \vec{E} = -\mu \frac{\partial \vec{H}}{\partial t}.$$

Collecting equations derived throughout the previous discussion,

$$(1)\ \nabla \cdot \vec{D} = \rho$$

$$(2)\ \nabla \cdot \vec{B} = 0$$

$$(3)\ \nabla \times \vec{E} = -\frac{\partial \vec{B}}{\partial t} = -\mu \frac{\partial \vec{H}}{\partial t}$$

$$(4)\ \nabla \times \vec{H} = \vec{J}_\mathrm{C} + \vec{J}_\mathrm{d}$$

$$= \sigma_\mathrm{c} \vec{E} + \varepsilon \frac{\partial \vec{E}}{\partial t}.$$

These are the most important relations in electromagnetic fields and constitute one of the most significant results in electrical engineering and physics. They are *Maxwell's equations.*

The material explained above is used to determine the electromagnetic fields necessary for producing the required values for a particular application. Having outlined the basic ideas of electromagnetic theory, it is now possible to understand more clearly the applications in psychiatry.

4.3 Vagus nerve stimulation (VNS)

The vagus nerve, labelled CNX, where X is the Roman number 10, is one of 12 pairs of cranial nerves (shown in figure 4.2) emanating from the brain stem not going through the spinal cord. Its terminal is in a structure in the brain stem called the *nucleus tractus solitarius.*

Upon leaving the medulla oblongata between the olive and the inferior cerebellar peduncle, the vagus nerve extends through the jugular foramen, then passes into the carotid sheath between the internal carotid artery and the internal jugular vein down to the neck, chest, and abdomen, where it contributes to the innervation of the viscera, reaching all the way to the colon. In addition, giving some output to various organs, the vagus nerve comprises between 80% and 90% of afferent nerves mostly

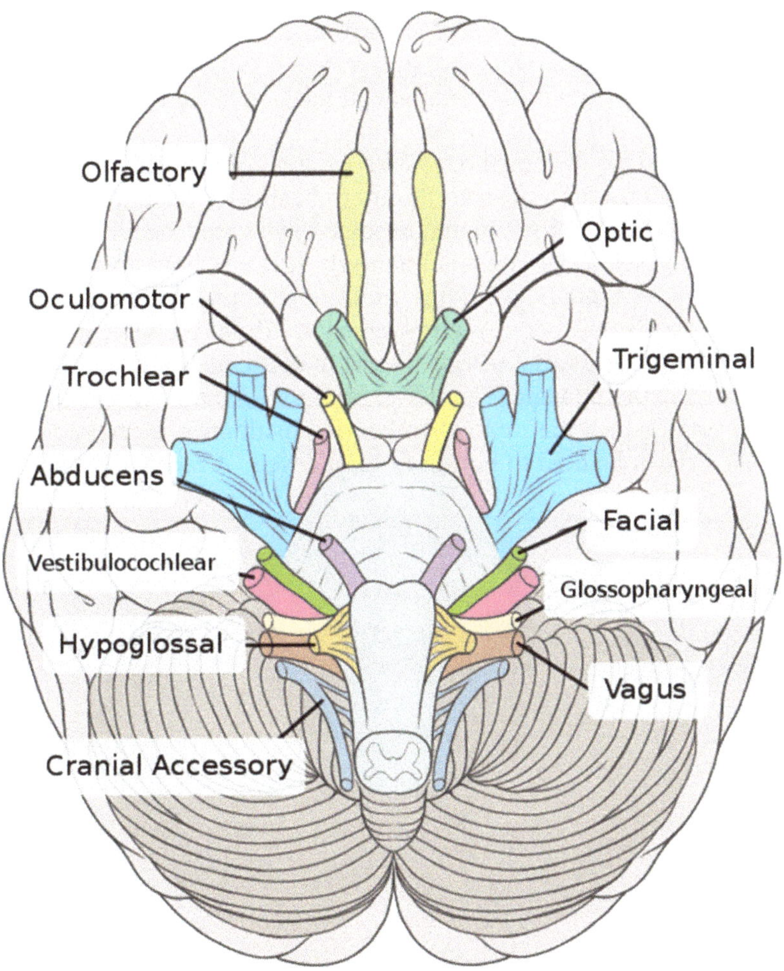

Figure 4.2. Cranial nerves including the vagus nerve [2, 3]. *Source*: Patrick J Lynch https://commons.wikimedia.org/wiki/file:brain_human_normal_inferior_view_withlabels_en.svg CC BY-SA 2.5.

conveying sensory information about the state of the body's organs to the central nervous system.

The right and left vagus nerves descend from the cranial vault through the jugular foramin, penetrating the carotid sheath between the internal and external carotid arteries, then passing posterolateral to the common carotid artery. The cell bodies of visceral afferent fibres of the vagus nerve are located bilaterally in the inferior ganglion of the vagus nerve (nodose ganglia) [3, 8] (figure 4.3).

The stimulation of the nerve is meant to inhibit the over-excitable neurons. An electric pulse generator is implanted in the chest and sends stimulating pulses to the vagus nerve which in turn sends signals to the brain that reduce severe chronic depression in some patients. The pulses can be programmed with typical properties being 2 mA amplitude and 250 μs width with a frequency of 20–30 Hz. The pulses are applied for 20 s, periodically every 5 min. Initially this technique was used to treat epilepsy but has later been used to tackle depression despite the lack of knowledge as to how it really works. However, limited success has been seen in severely depressed patients who did not respond to drugs and the only other alternative was electroconvulsive therapy with the associated risk of amnesia, which horrified candidates.

A common goal of the methods used to treat depression is to inhibit the reabsorption of serotonin, a neurotransmitter chemical. This implies that the goal is to increase the level of serotonin and in some other cases the release of inhibitory neurotransmitters such as gamma aminobutyric acid and norepinephrine. This will tone down the over-excitability of the brain and improve the pathology of the corresponding parts in the body. With psychoactive drugs the same goal is achieved by a chemical but of course this affects the entire brain, not just the parts thought to be responsible for the ailment. The device technologies aim to target the specific areas of the brain which are thought to be malfunctioning. Depression is another area where VNS can be used to boost serotonin levels. A recent development is the

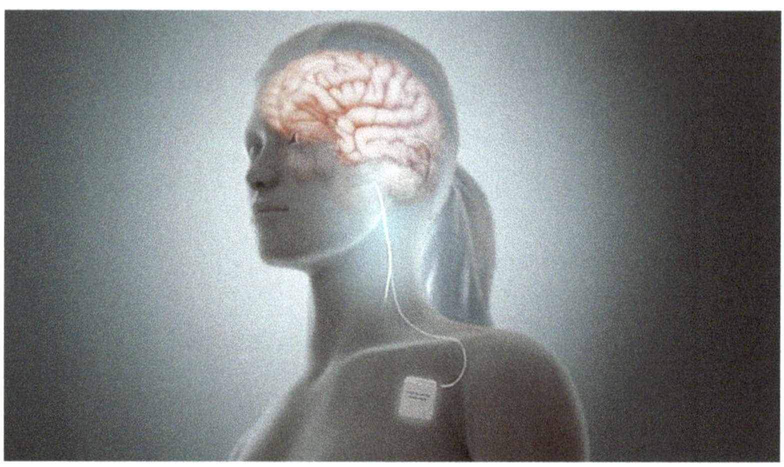

Figure 4.3. Vagus nerve stimulation using an electronic pulse generator [4]. *Source*: Manu5 https://commons.wikimedia.org/wiki/File:Vagus_nerve_stimulation.jpg CC BY-SA 4.0.

design of non-invasive vagus nerve stimulators. This has been an exceedingly difficult engineering problem. In order to reach the nerve using pulses from the outside of the body, the pulses must achieve two contradictory properties. First, the brain responses to VNS are frequency dependent. The nerve must receive a pulse with the low frequency of about 25 Hz, the direct transmission of which would, on their way, have to pass through a few centimetres of flesh which has a high resistance and is rich in pain receptors. To avoid the pain the external frequency is chosen as a burst of 5000 Hz and is *internally* down-converted to the 25 Hz. The solution to this problem is to recognise that the skin acts like a high pass filter which blocks low frequencies and lets higher frequencies pass, and then the 5000 Hz are down-converted by the *nerve cells themselves* to the 25 Hz required to stimulate the vagus nerve and propagate to the brain. The external high frequency loses only about half of its strength and does not affect the pain receptors in the skin.

VNS can be also used in a number of other neurological ailments. In epilepsy it tones down the excitability of the brain leading to reduced electrical storms associated with epileptic seizures. It can also reduce the over-excitability in the brain leading to migraine and cluster headaches. Another application is to combine certain sound tones with VNS to reduce the ringing in the ears leading to tinnitus. Stroke victims can benefit from combining this technique with specific body movements to speed up the relearning process of these movements.

Other non-neurological areas are heart failure, obesity, diabetes, Crohn's disease, and rheumatoid arthritis.

4.4 Repetitive transcranial magnetic stimulation (rTMS)

The prefrontal cortex is mainly responsible for decision making but the neural activities in this region have been found to be abnormal in people suffering from depression and connected with mood regulation structures deep in the brain. This method is seen as an alternative to electroconvulsive therapy. It consists of the following steps where all the quantities are time varying with the given typical amplitudes (figure 4.4):

a. A powerful electromagnet is positioned over the prefrontal cortex which uses windings with 1 kV applied.
b. The voltage produces a current of 8 kA.
c. The current gives rise to a strong magnetic field of about 2 T.

According to the exposition on electromagnetism discussed earlier in this chapter, the time-varying magnetic field induces an electric current in the neurons. The relation is given by the fourth Maxwell's equation. It produces a current in the prefrontal cortex activating the neurons. The resulting pulsating current passes through a region of a few cubic centimetres and is maintained for a few minutes per day over weeks. It has a long-term effect on the neuron activities.

The use of this method is, at best, semi-empirical because we do not have an accurate model of the *interaction* between the magnetic field and the neurons. In the next chapter we shall see how the interaction between the external applied field and

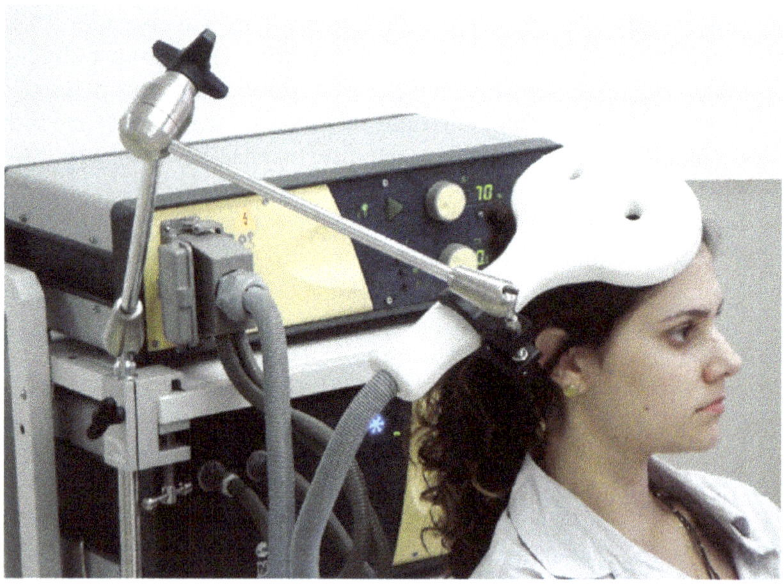

Figure 4.4. Repetitive transcranial magnetic stimulation [5]. *Source*: Baburov https://commons.wikimedia.org/wiki/File:Neuro-ms.png CC BY-SA 4.0.

neural tissue can be calculated using Maxwell's equations and assess the accuracy of the result.

A complete knowledge of the risks and long-term side effects is still lacking. The problem of accuracy has been addressed by incorporating magnetic resonance maps of the patients' brains to guide the application of the current to the required location in the brain.

4.5 Magnetic seizure therapy [1]

This is really a magnetic version of electroconvulsive therapy. A powerful electromagnet induces a high frequency electric current in a small part of the brain until it sparks a seizure. It is hoped that it will have the same effect on treating depression while avoiding the problem of memory loss associated with electroconvulsive therapy which triggers a seizure in a wide area of the brain. Nevertheless, the magnetic version requires anaesthetic and careful monitoring for weeks. Little is known about side effects.

4.6 Transcranial direct current stimulation (tDCS) [1]

A device drives a small dc current of the order of 1 mA through the prefrontal lobe for a minute per day for several weeks and it alters the neuron activity in the long term. It is rather simple, but the idea is the same as the repetitive transcranial stimulation and seeks to excite the neurons increasing the propagation of signals. In this case it creates a biasing current via electrodes raising the probability of propagation.

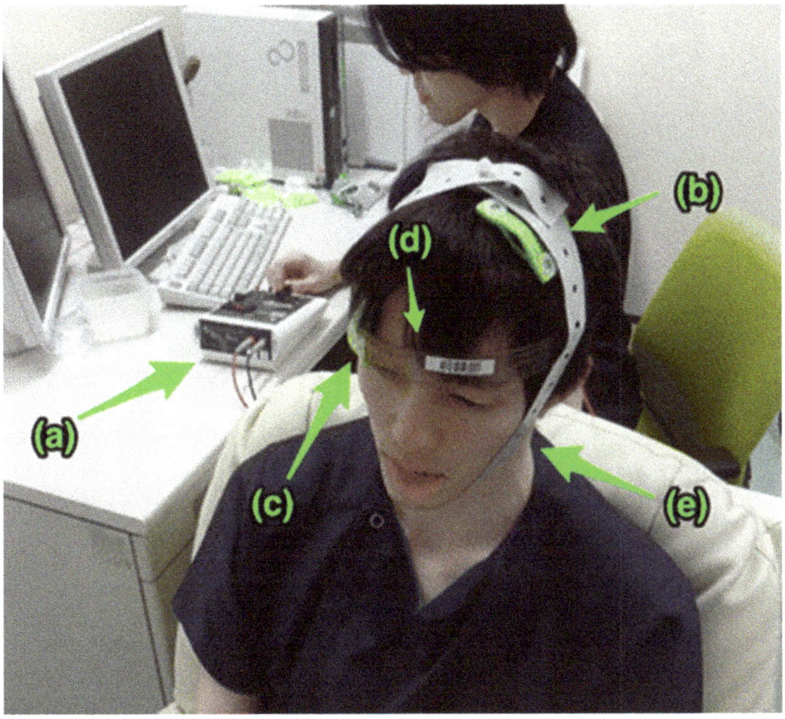

Figure 4.5. Transcranial direct current stimulation [6]. *Source*: Yokoi and Sumiyoshi https://commons.wikimedia.org/wiki/File:TDCS_administration.gif CC BY-SA 4.0.

With reference to figure 4.5 for tDCS administration anodal (a), anodal (b), and cathodal (c) electrodes with 35 cm^2 size are put on the F3 and right supraorbital regions, respectively. A head strap (d) is used for convenience and reproducibility, and a rubber band (e) for reducing resistance.

4.7 Deep brain stimulation (DBS) [7]

This is a more drastic approach reserved for patients as a last resort. Electrodes are inserted deep in the brain which receive electric pulses from a pulse generator in the chest. These switch off neurons located within a few millimetres from the electrodes. It can treat severe depression by interrupting malfunctioning neural networks responsible for the condition. Some effects are almost instantaneous because of the accurate targeting, but it requires surgery to insert the electrodes deep inside the brain and running wires under the skin in the neck to connect the electrodes to a device implanted in the chest (figure 4.6).

Early uses of this method were to reduce the tremors of Parkinson's disease (PD) [2]. In this case, the pulses are 3–5 V in amplitude with 100 Hz frequency. The pulses suppress the neuron activity in the vicinity of the electrodes in a manner of a 'reversible tenable' surgery since the device can be turned on and off to bring back the neuron activity. This, of course, is a conjecture or wishful thinking since the

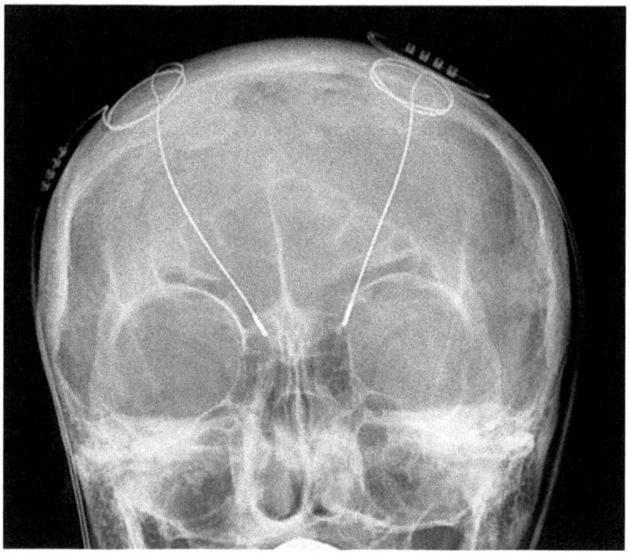

Figure 4.6. Deep brain stimulation [7]. *Source*: Hellerhoff https://commons.wikimedia.org/wiki/File:Tiefe_Hirnstimulation_-_Sonden_RoeSchaedel_ap.jpg CC BY-SA 3.0.

mechanism is not precisely known. The technique has also been tried for treatment of obsessive compulsive disorder (OCD) and this has actually been its first use in psychiatry which has replaced the earlier method of destroying a small part of the brain. DBS is used to manage some of the symptoms of PD that cannot be adequately controlled with medications. It is recommended for people who have PD with motor fluctuations and tremor inadequately controlled by medication, or for those who are intolerant to medication, as long as they do not have severe neuropsychiatric problems. Four areas of the brain have been treated with neural stimulators in PD. These are the globus pallidus internus, thalamus, subthalamic nucleus, and the pedunculopontine nucleus. However, most DBS surgeries in routine practice target either the globus pallidus internus, or the subthalamic nucleus.

DBS of the globus pallidus internus reduces uncontrollable shaking movements called dyskinesias. This enables a patient to take adequate quantities of medications (in particular levodopa), thus leading to better control of symptoms. DBS of the subthalamic nucleus directly reduces symptoms of Parkinson's. This enables a decrease in the dose of anti-parkinsonian medications. DBS has been used experimentally in treating adults with severe Tourette's syndrome that does not respond to conventional treatment. Despite widely publicised early successes, DBS remains a highly experimental procedure for the treatment of Tourette's, and more research is needed to determine whether the long-term benefits outweigh the risks. The procedure is well tolerated, but complications include short battery life, abrupt symptom worsening upon cessation of stimulation, hypomanic or manic conversion, and the significant time and effort involved in optimising stimulation parameters [7]. The procedure is invasive and expensive and requires long-term expert care.

4.8 Digital psychiatry

The present wide-spread use of smart phones, health apps, and wearables can be adapted to create a useful and accessible area of psychiatry which covers both diagnosis and treatment. In many countries the health system is cumbersome and slow and cannot provide the necessary care for psychiatric patients.

The use of a smart wearable either as a standalone device or in conjunction with a smart phone has offered immense possibilities in the diagnosis and treatment of depression, schizophrenia, and other disorders.

- The devices can use WiFi to track patient location when GPS is unavailable. They can also tag certain sites such as gymnasia or bars which the patient may frequent.
- Bluetooth and near field communication (NFC) can track physical proximity to other devices in order to evaluate social relationships or appointments with the treating psychiatrist.
- Heart rate and temperature sensors on the devices can detect nervous system activities and mood changes which may be associated with certain conditions such as increased levels of anxiety.
- GPS can track social behavioural patterns which would be helpful in assessing many disorders.
- Accelerometers and gyroscopes track physical activities and tremors which are also useful in assessing many disorders.
- The camera can track facial expressions which may reveal mood changes and anxiety levels in addition to eye movements which may reveal side effects of medication.
- The touch screen can track response time and task completion duration which would be useful in assessing cognition.
- Proximity sensors would help in many disorders by evaluating social behaviour.
- Sleep tracking applications can detect sleep disorders and evaluate the effect of medications.
- Smart spectacles have been used to read facial expressions and provide social clues to autistic children.
- Wearable cameras combined with software can detect emotions in order to give social cues in real time to track responses for later analysis by the therapist.

The collection of data using the wearable and smart phone applications can all be combined not only for diagnosis and monitoring but also for treatment. For example, sensors can be embodied in pills which are ingested to detect the level of stomach acid indicating whether the pill has been taken by the patient then sends a signal to a wearable device which in turn sends the information via Bluetooth to a smart phone or in the case of a standalone wearable directly to the treating psychiatrist. Of course, not all treatments rely on medication, instead therapy sessions can be held over a smart phone or a computer. Virtual reality tools are now in use to reduce the delusions that are characteristic of some disorders such as schizophrenia or autism. Along similar lines, artificial intelligence (AI) psychotherapists can be designed in the form of mobile telephone apps or wearables to respond in emergencies which occur randomly throughout the day or night. Some details are given in [9].

4.9 Conclusion

Electronic brain stimulation techniques which can be used in psychiatry have been discussed. The background for the techniques in electromagnetic field theory has been summarised offering the opportunity of a better understanding of the underlying engineering principles.

One can envisage that when drug therapy fails, the use of these methods may be offered according to the following order of increased degree of invasiveness:

a. Transcranial direct current stimulation.
b. Repetitive transcranial magnetic stimulation.
c. Seizure therapy.
d. Deep brain stimulation and vagus nerve stimulation which require surgery.

Clearly the success of these methods requires close cooperation between electronic engineers, neuroscientists, clinical neurologists, and neurosurgeons.

The development of smart phones and wearable devices with sensors and dedicated apps have created the new discipline of *digital psychiatry* which allows the diagnosis, monitoring, and therapy of psychological disorders.

References

[1] Moore S K 2006 Psychiatry's shocking new tools *IEEE Spectr.* **43** 18–25 March

[2] Lynch P J 2009 File:Brain human normal inferior view with labels en.svg *Wikimedia Commons* https://commons.wikimedia.org/wiki/File:Brain_human_normal_inferior_view_with_labels_en.svg

[3] Vagus nerve *Wikipedia* https://en.wikipedia.org/wiki/Vagus_nerve

[4] Manu5 2018 File:Vagus nerve stimulation.jpg *Wikimedia Commons* https://commons.wikimedia.org/wiki/File:Vagus_nerve_stimulation.jpg

[5] Baburov 2015 File:Neuro-ms.png *Wikimedia Commons* https://commons.wikimedia.org/wiki/File:Neuro-ms.png

[6] Yokoi and Sumiyoshi 2015 File:TDCS administration.gif *Wikimedia Commons* https://commons.wikimedia.org/wiki/File:TDCS_administration.gif

[7] Hellerhoff 2011 File:Tiefe Hirnstimulation - Sonden RoeSchaedel ap.jpg *Wikimedia Commons* https://commons.wikimedia.org/wiki/File:Tiefe_Hirnstimulation_-_Sonden_RoeSchaedel_ap.jpg

[8] Johns P 2014 *Clinical Neuroscience* (London: Churchill Livingstone Elsevier)

[9] Torous J 2017 Digital psychiatry *IEEE Spectr.* **54** 45–50 July

IOP Publishing

Electronic Engineering for Neuromedicine

Hussein Baher

Chapter 5

Neural engineering: merging neuroscience with engineering

5.1 Introduction

From the previous chapters, it is clear that a new discipline can be formulated which combines engineering with neuroscience. This is *neural engineering* [1]. Indeed, this field has emerged as a natural outcome of the collaboration between engineers and neuroscientists to study the nervous system and apply the results in neuromedicine. In this chapter we highlight further aspects of this hybrid field by giving a number of its applications. We mainly point out some important results, representative examples, and indicate the publications where the details may be found.

5.2 Scanning and imaging techniques [1, 2]

Medical scanning and imaging techniques, in particular ultrasound (US), computer tomography (CT), and magnetic resonance imaging (MRI), have transformed medical practice in general and neuromedicine in particular because they allow the study and diagnosis of brain problems in a completely non-invasive manner.

In general, there are four types of medical image:

i. *Sonographic*. An ultrasound image is created which uses ultrasound waves and very often together with the *Doppler effect*.
ii. *Topographic*. This represents a part of the surface of the body and is usually formed using visible light.
iii. *Projection*. This is formed by the interaction of radiation, penetrating the body along predetermined paths, with specific regions. An example is the x-ray or Röntgen image.
iv. *Tomographic image*. This gives the spatial distribution of the interaction of radiation with tissue in a localised thin slice through the body. The significance of CT technology was recognised in 1979, with the Nobel Prize being awarded to the electrical engineer Godfrey Hounsfield and the physicist Alan Cormack for the 'development of computer-assisted tomography'.

In all cases, the quality of the image is judged by two parameters: contrast and resolution.

Contrast is determined by one of several factors:

a. The nature of the interaction of the radiation with the tissue material, for example via partial absorption.
b. The nature of the interaction of the radiation with the tissue structure, for example via reflection.
c. The differentiated accumulation of an indicator substance, such as iodine in the case of x-rays, gadolinium for MRI, microbubbles for ultrasound, and radionuclides for scintigraphy.

Resolution is defined as (a) spatial-contrast in terms of the modulation transfer characteristic (output–input relation) of the imager, and (b) temporal resolution defined as the exposure time needed to complete the scan of a single image and the frame rate of the sequence of images. Specifically, in tomography we speak of *voxels* which are the three-dimensional counterparts of *pixels*.

5.3 Electromagnetic radiation and wave propagation

The solution of Maxwell's equations under given boundary conditions gives rise to the phenomena of wave propagation and electromagnetic radiation. This means that the presence of time-varying electric and magnetic fields leads to waves that propagate between various points in a medium. The waves have frequencies of propagation dependent on the medium and sources of the electric and magnetic sources. The theoretical lower limit is Planck's length of about 1.616×10^{-35} m while the theoretical upper limit is the size of the Universe.

The electromagnetic frequency spectrum covers the range of frequencies of electromagnetic radiation and their respective wavelengths and photon energies. This range is from a fraction of a hertz to above 10^{25} Hz. This corresponds to wavelengths of a few kilometres to a fraction of an angstrom (one angstrom = 10^{-10} m). The spectrum is divided into the ranges of radio waves (RF), microwaves, infrared, visible light, ultraviolet (UV), x-rays, and gamma rays. These types differ in the way they are generated and the way they interact with matter. High UV, x-ray, and gamma rays are *ionising radiations*, since the corresponding high-energy photons cause chemical reactions which ionise atoms.

5.4 Magnetic resonance imaging (MRI)

5.4.1 Resonance

Resonance is a property of systems containing energy storage components. Suppose we have a series combination of an inductor which stores magnetic energy, a capacitor which stores electric energy, and a resistor which dissipates energy. Then a voltage is applied to the combination. The impedance as a function of frequency ω is

$$Z = R + j\omega L - \frac{1}{j\omega C},$$

which reaches the minimum value R at a frequency of

$$\omega_0 = 1/\sqrt{LC},$$

which means that for any small voltage the current would be V/R and if R is small the current would be very large, theoretically infinite for $R = 0$, and we say that at this frequency the circuit is at series resonance. Resonances produce peaks in the response and these peaks depend on the values of L, C, and R which are properties of the medium. Thus, if we excite a medium with a frequency-varying source the medium will show characteristics which will define many properties of the medium. Mechanical and biological systems also exhibit resonance properties. In mechanical systems L and C will have their counterparts as the mass and stiffness, respectively. R would be the friction resulting in energy loss or dissipation.

5.4.2 Dipoles

Positive and negative electric charges exist separately in nature, for example an electron has a negative charge while a proton has a positive one, and they can exist independently. We come across the concept of a *dipole* very often in electromagnetic fields and hence in neuromedicine. An electric dipole is simply a system consisting of a positive charge $+Q$ and a negative one $-Q$ separated by a distance L. The electric dipole moment is a vector of magnitude QL in the direction from $-Q$ towards $+Q$. For a small separation at the atomic level the dipole is given the symbol $\vec{p}$ and is treated as a single element existing at a well-defined point for which the electric field at a relatively large distance can be calculated as if pointing from the dipole itself to the point.

Now, *magnetic poles* do not exist independently in nature, rather as magnetic *dipoles*. A magnetic dipole is a north pole and a south pole separated by a distance. In electromagnetism the source of magnetic fields is the current carrying conductor and since currents need closed paths to exist, a current carrying loop generates a magnetic field analogous to a dipole or a magnet (composed of north and south poles existing together) which is a vector whose direction is normal to the plane of the loop and obeys the right-hand screw rule. Its magnitude depends on the circumference of the loop and the value of the current. A current is defined as the motion of electric charge so that a particle which rotates or spins about its axis with an angular velocity has spin and acts as a magnetic dipole which is a basic magnetic element giving rise to a magnetic field. Elementary particles are regarded as point charges and as such there is no clear meaning to a spinning particle around an axis as the angular momentum of a particle moving around an axis. However, this is one of the wondrous assumptions of quantum mechanics and in particular the work of Wolfgang Pauli. An electron or a proton has a spin and has magnetic properties *as if* (in German this translates into *als ob*) it had an angular momentum in the classical sense. With the spin there is an associated magnetic dipole moment and a magnetic field.

The ideas of resonance, magnetic dipoles, spin, and magnetic fields are used together in MRI imaging in a non-invasive manner according to the following principles:

a. A spinning particle acts as a magnetic dipole with a moment as vector and produces a corresponding magnetic field.
b. Any system has natural or resonance frequencies at which the system either emits or absorbs energy.
c. Magnetic dipoles align in accordance with a strong applied magnetic field.
d. The change of state from alignment to misalignment releases energy at the natural frequencies of the system. This is due to the difference between the two energy levels of an ordered and a disordered system.

In MRI [1–3] the body is subjected to a strong magnetic field of the order of 1.5 T. The basic elements of a scanner are illustrated in figure 5.1. Each proton in the hydrogen atoms which, together with oxygen, make up the water content in the body has a *spin* (equivalent to rotation about an axis) of value (1/2) ($h/2\pi$) where h is Plank's constant. The proton is a positively charged particle. If it spins (or *acts* as a spinning particle in the mysterious assumptions of quantum mechanics) it is an

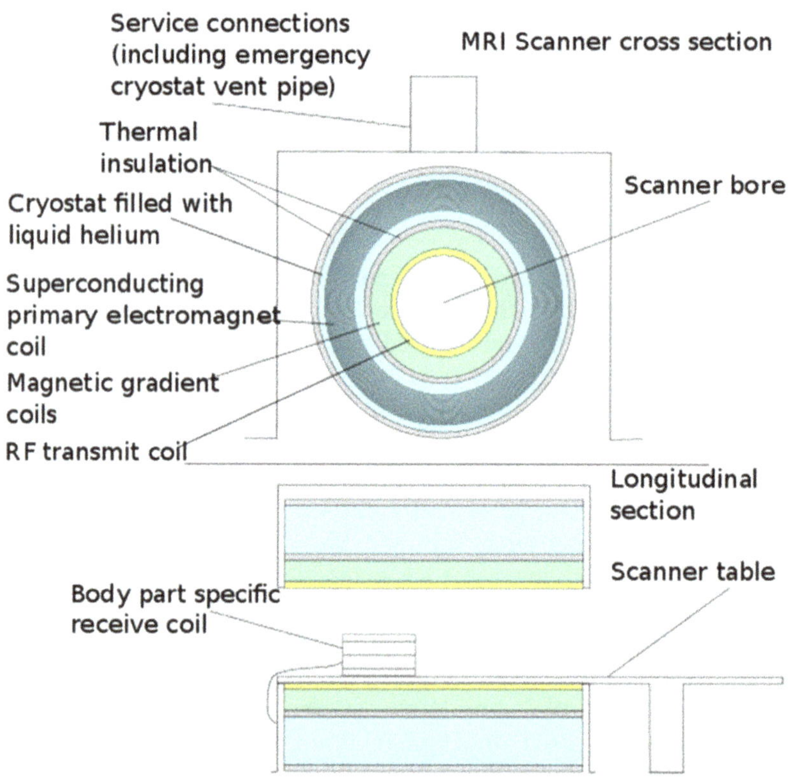

Figure 5.1. MRI scanner [5]. *Source*: ChumpusRex https://en.wikipedia.org/wiki/File:Mri_scanner_schematic_labelled.svg CC BY-SA 3.0.

effective moving charge, and this is the definition of an electric current, like a current carrying loop. This produces a magnetic field along its axis. Thus, the proton acts like a magnetic dipole with effective north and south poles. Therefore, the magnetic field aligns the protons in its direction, i.e. along the magnetic field lines. By a sequence of switching the magnetic field on and off in combination with an RF signal the protons are forced to return to their non-alignment state. This transition between the two states gives rise to an RF emission by the protons which in turn creates a characteristic pattern of the tissue in which the process takes place. This pattern provides the information about the nature of the tissue. Unlike x-rays, MR is a non-ionising radiation so it has no harmful effects. Due to the strength of the magnetic field which uses an electromagnet with windings, carrying high current values these should be made up of superconductors which need to be maintained at very low temperatures using liquid helium. Typical brain scans are shown in figures 5.2 and 5.3. More recently, low power MRI machines using field strengths as low as several micro- or milli-tesla have been in use and are useful in mobile MRI scanning units [4].

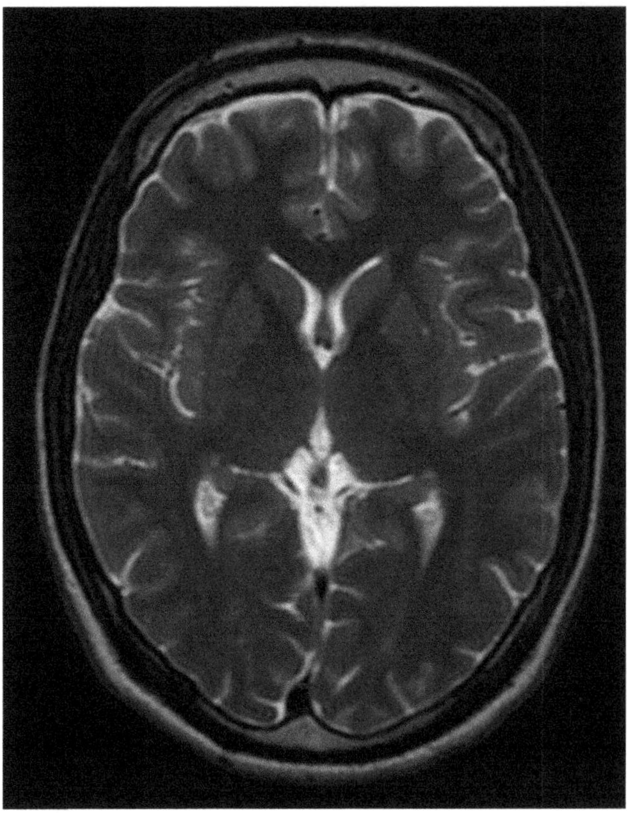

Figure 5.2. Typical normal MRI brain scan result [6]. *Source*: Novaksean https://commons.wikimedia.org/wiki/File:Normal_axial_T2-weighted_MR_image_of_the_brain.jpg CC BY-SA 4.0.

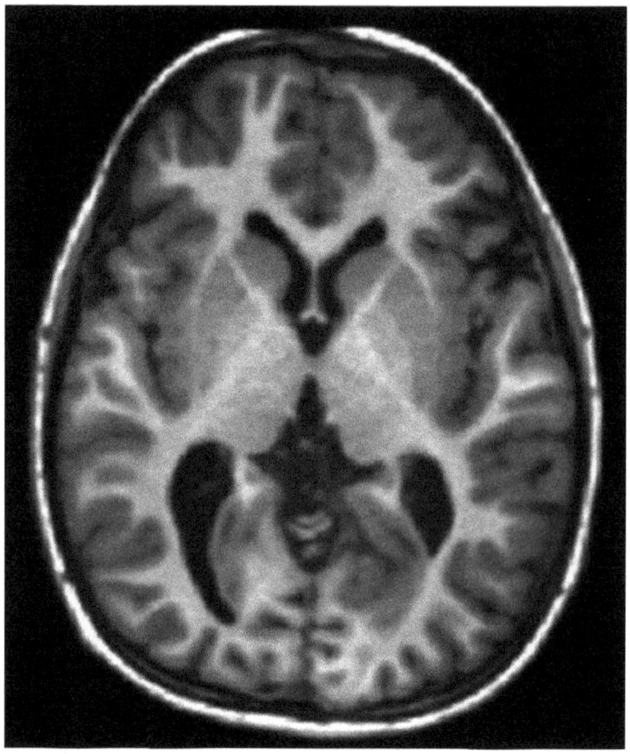

Figure 5.3. Typical normal MRI brain scan result [7]. *Source*: Mim.cis https://commons.wikimedia.org/wiki/File:T1-weighted-MRI.png Public Domain.

Magnetic resonance angiography (MRA) (figure 5.4) generates pictures of the arteries to evaluate them for stenosis (abnormal narrowing) or aneurysms (vessel wall dilatations, at risk of rupture). MRA is often used to evaluate the arteries of the neck and brain, thoracic and abdominal aorta, the renal arteries, and the legs. A variety of techniques can be used to generate the pictures, such as administration of a paramagnetic contrast agent (gadolinium).

Functional MRI (fMRI) observes the *activities* in the various regions of the brain under different stimuli. This has been of immense importance in understanding the different functions of the brain regions as they relate to motor and sensory functions as well as the very complex and illusory property of *cognition*.

5.5 Blood supply ultrasound Doppler scans

The upper limit of human audible sound frequencies is about 20 kHz. Ultrasound is above this value. Diagnostic imaging is used with ultrasound resulting in the technique known as *sonography*. This is achieved by sending pulses of ultrasound into the tissue using a probe. The reflection forms an echo from the tissue with different refractive properties and the result is recorded and displayed as an image. In the case of blood flow, the speed produces a Doppler effect (frequency change

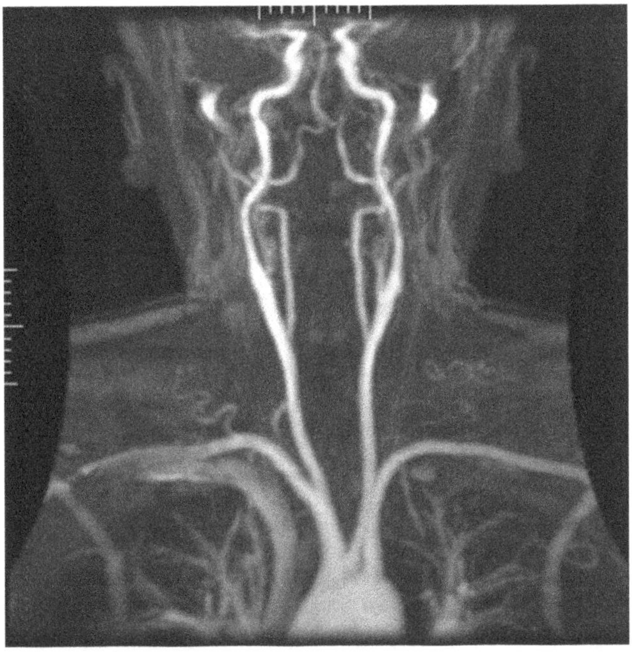

Figure 5.4. MRA [8]. *Source*: Ofir Glazer https://commons.wikimedia.org/wiki/File:Mra1.jpg CC BY-SA 3.0.

with speed of moving source object) which is used to measure the speed and hence the flow rate. The most common type of image is a B mode which is a function of brightness. It displays the acoustic impedance of a two-dimensional cross section of the tissue. US scanners provide images in real time so that the blood flow for example can be seen in real time and recorded. It can be also portable and does not use ionising radiation. These methods are much simpler than MRI and provide a quick and completely non-invasive study of the arteries supplying the blood to the brain.

The arterial blood supply to the brain comes from four arteries two of which are the two interior carotid arteries. The use of ultrasound methods to reveal the internal pathology of the carotid arteries has been of great help in the diagnosis of stenosis and brain strokes and the risks of such events in a completely non-invasive and safe way. This is illustrated in figures 5.5 and 5.6.

5.6 Interaction of electric fields with neural tissue [11]

In the central nervous systems neurons exist in an extracellular medium with a relatively low resistivity of the order of 80–300 Ω cm. In using electrodes for any purpose such as study, monitoring, excitation, or inhibition of neuronal signals, it is necessary to calculate the distribution of the electric field and voltage in the vicinity of the electrodes. As a first step, certain approximations are made. We are dealing with frequencies below 10 kHz so that we can make the assumption of *quasistatic*

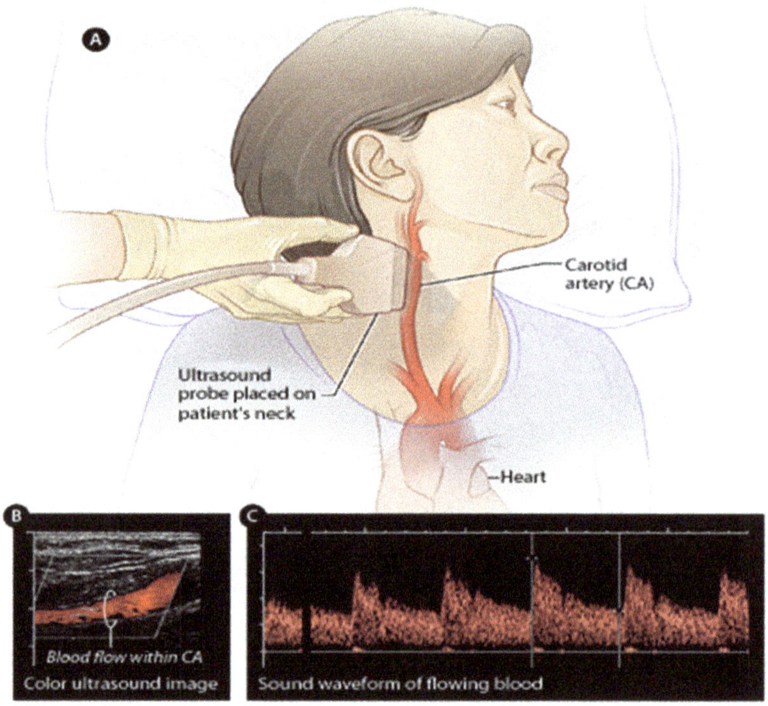

Figure 5.5. Carotid ultrasound [9]. *Source*: National Heart Lung and Blood Institute (NIH) https://commons.wikimedia.org/wiki/File:Carotid_ultrasound.jpg Public Domain.

fields. In this case, the time-varying terms in Maxwell's equations are neglected and Maxwell's equations can be reduced to

$$\nabla . \vec{J} = 0$$

$$\nabla . \vec{E} = \rho / \varepsilon$$

$$\vec{J} = \sigma E$$

$$\vec{E} = -\nabla V,$$

where $\vec{E}$ is the electric field intensity, $\vec{J}$ is the current density, σ is the conductivity of the medium, and ε is the permittivity of the medium. The simultaneous solution of these equations subject to the specific boundary conditions gives the distribution of the voltage and electric field throughout the medium. In our case of a number of n electrodes currying currents I_k we obtain the voltage at a point due to all the currents as

$$V = \frac{1}{4\pi\sigma} \sum_{k=1}^{n} I_k / r_k .$$

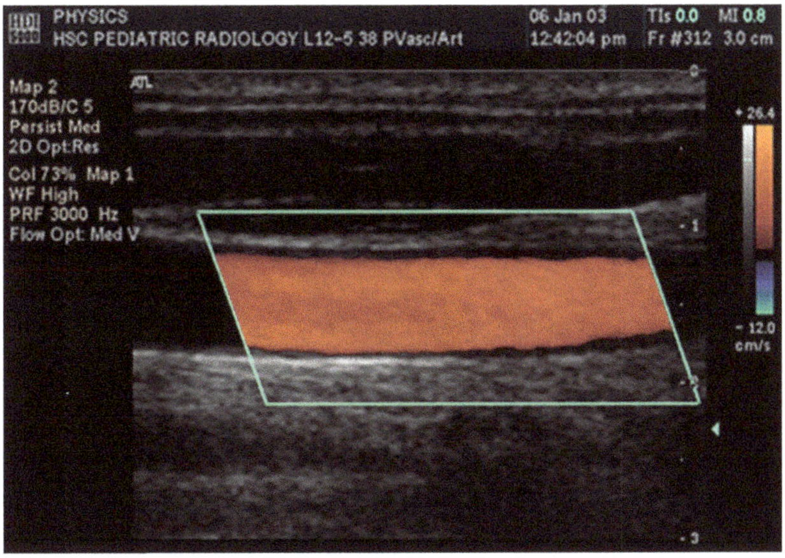

Figure 5.6. Blood flow in carotid artery [10]. *Source*: Drickey https://commons.wikimedia.org/wiki/File:ColourDopplerA.jpg CC BY-SA 2.5.

If we have two electrodes a distance d from each other the voltage difference between two points Δx apart in a uniform homogeneous medium which produces a resistance R between the two electrodes will be

$$\Delta V = -IR\Delta x/d.$$

This can be adapted for non-homogeneous media using numerical techniques such as finite element methods.

5.7 Application in epilepsy [11]

The above results can be applied to the suppression and control of epileptiform activity. In epilepsy a large number of neurons fire uncontrollably in a synchronised manner. The balance between excitation and inhibition is lost. It is relatively easy to envisage the mechanism of excitation of neurons by the application of electric fields. But using the fields to induce inhibition and desynchronisation of neurons is more difficult. Nevertheless, the mechanism of interaction in both excitation and inhibition is the same as explained in the previous section. We pursue this further to indicate how this may be used to suppress epileptiform activity and control the seizures or *ictal events*.

The current flow around the electrodes is governed by the equations of the above section. The current through the cell bodies can flow outwards causing depolarisation or inwards across the membrane causing hyperpolarisation. The effect can be modelled either analytically or numerically. The membrane voltage satisfies the following differential equation:

$$\gamma^2 \frac{\partial^2 V}{\partial x^2} - \beta \frac{\partial V}{\partial t} - V = -\gamma^2 \frac{\partial^2 V_{\text{ex}}}{\partial x^2},$$

where V is the transmembrane voltage and the so-called *space constant* γ of the membrane is given by

$$\gamma = 0.5\sqrt{\frac{R_{ms}D}{R_{as}}},$$

where R_{ms} is the specific resistance of the membrane, R_{as} is the axoplasmic specific resistance, D is the diameter of the dendrite, and β is the time constant of the membrane given by

$$\beta = R_m C_m.$$

These equations allow the calculation of the transmembrane voltage via the electrodes due to the application of the electric field.

We know that electric fields are generated endogenously by the nervous system, and they directly affect neural activity. Similarly, external applied electric fields can affect neural activity to cause either excitation or inhibition. In the control of epileptiform activity, the fields are used to restore the balance between the two activities or suppress the abnormal synchronised uncontrollable firing of neurons responsible for the seizure.

5.8 Electronics for paralysis [12]

In paralysis, the signals between the sensory and motor cortexes are interrupted. There are two ways of by-passing the damaged path and replacing it by an intact path which establishes the connection electronically:

i. In cases of total or severe paralysis, electrode arrays are implanted in the motor cortex, the sensory cortex, and the spinal cord. The person attempts to seize an object and the electrodes in the motor cortex pick up the neural signals generated as the person imagines moving arm and hand. The signals are decoded by an artificial intelligence (AI) powered processor which sends nerve stimulation instructions to an electrode pad on the arm. This passes back to the sensory cortex and the person feels the object he is holding and adjusts the grip. Another electrode array is placed in the spinal cord which stimulates the spinal nerves with the objective of promoting growth and regeneration. This implant-based system is, of course, invasive.
ii. In milder cases of partial loss of movement a wearable-based system may be used. This method places a patch on the arm which registers biometric signals as the person attempts to use his hand. These are naturally noisy signals which are decoded by the AI processor which sends nerve stimulation to the same arm patch. The electronics needed here are quite sophisticated since the signals are stochastic and noisy.

5.9 Artificial silicon retina [13]

The retina is a complex network of neural sensors. Designing an electronic approximation of the retina can be used for modelling purposes. In the human eye the retina contains millions of neurons performing image sensing, data smoothing, feature extraction, and dynamic processing.

The outer plexiform layer of the retina contains three major types of cell:

i. Photoreceptors which are transducers converting light into electric signals.
ii. Horizontal cells providing spatial-temporal smoothing of the signals from the photoreceptors. Smoothing is the term describing a type of filtering of stochastic signals.
iii. Bipolar cells which process the signals from the above types.

For simulation of the retina, cellular neural networks were introduced. These are simple repetitive structures capable of realisation in VLSI form while imitating specific neural functions. The term *cellular* means that the cell communicates only with the neighbouring cells. They are continuous time dynamic parallel processors capable of many image processing functions such as noise removal, corner detection, hole filling, and shadowing. The implementation uses microelectronic or nano-electronic devices (of dimensions of the order of 10^{-9} m). An example of such implementations was given in [13] using *neuron bipolar junction transistors* which are particularly suitable for realisation of so-called large *neighbourhood cellular networks*. They are capable of realising the three major cell types of the retina giving a useful degree of approximation. In medical applications the silicon retina would be implanted in place of the dysfunctional retina or a part of it. The image processing part can also be on the same silicon chip and the entire integrated circuits is powered by a photovoltaic cell using the input to the eye from light reflected from the outside objects as well as direct light (figure 5.7).

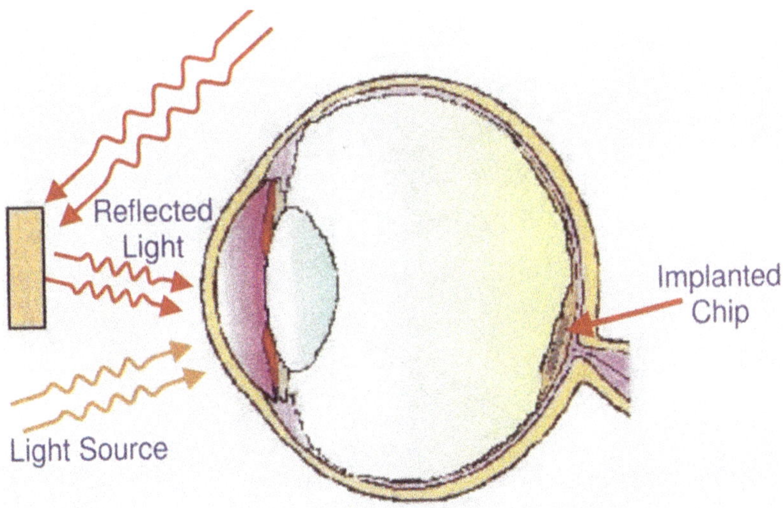

Figure 5.7. Artificial silicon retina. Reproduced with permission from [13]. Copyright 2001 IEEE.

5.10 Cochlear implant [14]

Sensorineural hearing loss (SNHL) is caused by a problem in the inner ear or sensory organ or the vestibulocochlear nerve. It can affect parts or all of the frequency spectrum. But in all cases, it is permanent. In moderate to profound cases, cochlear transplants have been in use for decades. This is meant to bypass the natural peripheral auditory system and stimulates the auditory nerve. The conventional apparatus consists of two parts, internal and external. The external device consists of microphones which convert the sound into electrical signals, filters and digital signal processing (DSP) circuits to select the band containing speech and digitise the result. This is then fed into an RF antenna which transmits the signal to the internal implant. This is placed surgically into the cochlea and receives the external processed signal using another antenna. The output stimulates the cochlear auditory nerve. The neural signals are then processed by the brain as in the natural hearing mechanism. Essentially, this arrangement by-passes most of the peripheral auditory system in favour of the electronic circuits contained in both the external and internal parts. More recently, attempts have been made to create an all-in-one device which contains both parts and constitutes a single internal implant which is of course totally invisible externally with a reduced risk of damage (figure 5.8).

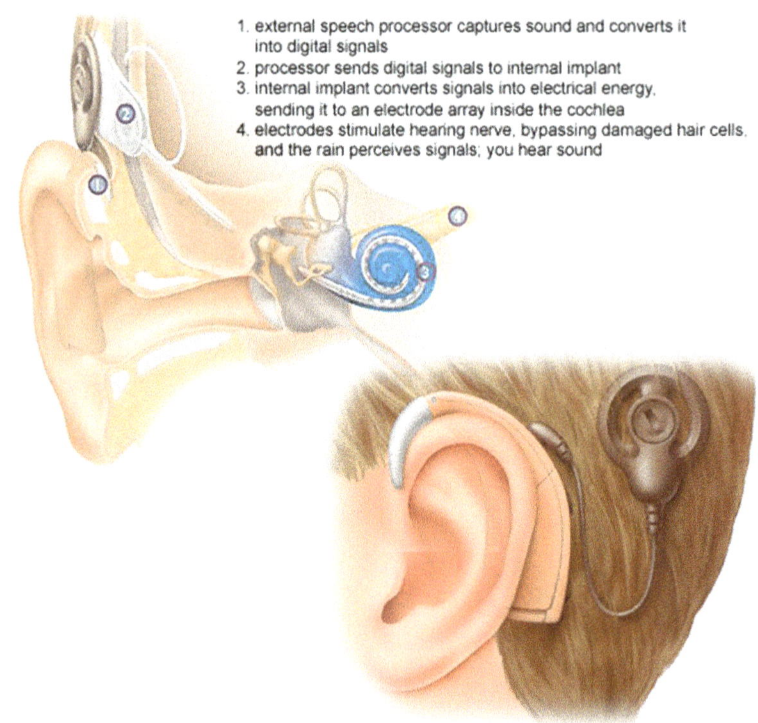

Figure 5.8. Cochlear implant [14]. *Source*: BC Family Hearing https://commons.wikimedia.org/wiki/File:Cochlear-implant.jpg CC BY-SA 4.0.

5.11 Electronic skin [15, 16]

The skin is the largest organ, functioning as an interface between the brain and the external world and containing a large number of sensors. Early research in developing an electronic version of the human skin was centred on use with robots, creating a flexible mesh and wrapping it around a robotic hand. Later attention moved to applying it directly to the human body. This could be used to monitor medical conditions or to design more sensitive and realistic prosthetics. The problems that were to be tackled involved the creation of highly flexible microelectronic circuits which can be wrapped around the body parts and joints while adapting to the soft human body. The need has arisen for electronic circuits which can bend around joints and have good mechanical properties. Unfortunately, conventional microelectronic circuits are generally constructed on rigid substrates such as silicon and glass. For an electronic skin we need electronics that can be bent, rolled, folded, and crumpled. Much progress has been made using thin film transistors which can be made of semiconductors deposited in thin layers, such as amorphous silicon or organic semiconductors. As substrates, materials such as ultrathin glass and plastic films can be used. Using these techniques E-skin has been constructed that is both flexible and stretchable.

5.12 Restoring the sense of touch [17]

Conventional prosthetics tend to be crude and not quite capable of endowing the user with the sensitive touch necessary for realistic usage. New prosthetics endowed with haptics allow the wearer to combine motor functions with a sense of connection. For example, in the case of a person with a missing hand, electrodes implanted in the wearer's arm make contact with the nerves at 20 locations. Stimulation of the nerve fibres creates a realistic sensation perceived as coming from the missing hand. For example, the stimulation of one spot produces a sensation in the palm while stimulating another produces a sensation in the thumb. The resulting sensations combined with the motor function of a conventional prosthetic can result in better control over the prosthetic hand.

There are varying degrees of invasiveness in this procedure. The least invasive of these inserts the electrodes in the muscles surrounding the nerve or wraps them around the axon, while a more invasive procedure inserts the electrodes in the nerves. An ambitious goal is to simulate the emotional content of the sense of touch which is essential in establishing the human bond.

5.13 Robo surgeon [18]

Performing operations in remote areas via a communication channel between the surgeon and patient using a robotic set-up is possible. It combines various areas of electronic engineering such as robotics, computer communications, Internet, microwave engineering, satellite communications, and cable and wireless transmission. These are integrated to allow the performance of a surgical procedure at a distance.

5.14 Electro-optic brain therapies [19]

Optogenetics uses light for the selective stimulation of neurons in the cortex. It has been used to monitor and control individual neurons in living tissue in mice, with future potential applications in humans. According to one method, the simulation technique is synchronised with electrophysiological recordings to produce what is called a closed loop. This allows the possible regulation and repair of neural microcircuits. The technique involves a number of components:

i. An optrode, a device for sensing biopotentials and producing light signals, e.g. the combination of electrodes and optical fibres. This device senses the low-voltage electrical activities of the brain on several channels which are digitised.
ii. A neuro-recording interface device which records the signals in (i).
iii. A neural signal processor which connects the results above with the next device.
iv. A controller. This closes the loop between the above results and the following stage.
v. An optical stimulator which produces the light signals for the stimulation of the specific neurons.

5.15 Neural prosthetics [20]

A major problem in electronic engineering for neuroscience is to design electronic circuits which can *speak* to neural cells in a language they can understand. This is essential in repairing damaged or diseased parts of the nervous system which may be achieved by replacing the damaged parts by prosthetics which in turn can replace the higher thought processes lost to illness or damage.

This is a very different problem from that of designing an artificial retina to replace a damaged one or that of a cochlear implant to bypass the peripheral auditory system or stimulating the sense of touch discussed above. In the case of designing a neural prosthetic to replace damaged neurons we attempt to *replace cognitive functions with microelectronic circuits* with inputs and outputs capable of communicating with other parts of the brain in the same manner as the biological damaged parts did. One such approach is to replace the neurons in the computational parts of the brains by implantable microelectronic silicon neurons which perform the same functions. These neural implants would transmit and receive computations to and from other parts of the brain.

It has been recognised that a successful neural microelectronic neural prosthetic implant must satisfy the following conditions:

- It must be truly biomimetic, i.e. the neuron models must realistically simulate the properties of biological neurons.
- The neuron models must be simulated in a collective environment of neurons not in isolation, i.e. as physiological and psychological systems.
- The implant must be capable of a high degree of miniaturisation, and due to the nature of the nervous system the microcircuits will ultimately operate in

mixed analog and digital modes (or more accurately in continuous and discrete modes).
- The implant must be capable of communication with the existing biological neurons bidirectionally, i.e. transmit and receive information. In principle this should not be problematic since both artificial and biological neurons use electric signals to communicate.
- The prosthetic must be personalisable, i.e. adaptable to the person's special needs and circumstances.
- The power requirement for operating the prosthetic must be considered. This is particularly important since the inner parts of the brain in which the prosthetic would be implanted are temperature sensitive.

5.16 Treatment of long Covid using electrical stimulation [21]

After recovery from the corona virus illness, some patients continue to suffer from neurological complaints such as brain fog, memory difficulties, reading difficulties, and extreme fatigue. Some neurologists tried electrical stimulation of the brain by passing low electric currents through the skull into the cortex. These symptoms have been named post-acute sequelae of SARS-CoV-2 infection (PASC). Not only does it produce neurological problems but it is also associated with heart palpitations and breathing problems. As discussed earlier, neurostimulation involves electrical stimulation of the brain or peripheral nerves. Due to the previous experience in other areas, the emergence of the long Covid symptoms suggested trying the same idea in this case also. The same technique of transcranial direct current stimulation discussed for the control of epilepsy in chapter 4 was tried to control the symptoms of long Covid. Also, vagus nerve stimulation (VNS) through the ear was tried using a portable home device. Some patients reported a reduction in the brain fog, depression, memory lapses, and mood swings associated with long Covid. It is not yet known why if at all this method is helpful. Some presumption is that the tDCS enhances brain plasticity which, as explained earlier, signifies the ability to form new connections between neurons. This leads to rehabilitation after injury. Also, if the immune system has developed problems, vagus nerve stimulation may help as has been shown in previous cases of overactivity of the immune system. These are early days yet for a firm understanding of the trial results.

5.17 Eavesdropping on the brain [22]

The brain is a highly complex network containing over 8.6×10^{10} neurons. The quest for having complete access to this network of electric switches has been one of the main areas of neural engineering. Viewed from an electronic engineer's perspective this has been a very difficult problem. We need to access *every signal from every neuron* which, although electrical in nature, exists in a gelatinous material. A digital probe is needed that is long enough to reach any part of the brain while being so thin as to pose no hazard to the cells. Recent results have shown that a neural implant with 10^4 electrodes is possible using a network of *neuropixels* which are essentially micrometre-size electrodes in direct contact with the neurons. This is a good example of the cooperation of microelectronic engineers and neuroscientists. For a review of these new innovations the reader may consult [22].

5.18 Magnetoencephalography (MEG) using quantum sensors [23]

The magnetic fields produced by the currents in the brain can be detected using quantum sensors. This allows the brain activities to be analysed in a non-invasive manner analogous to EEG but using the *magnetic effects* of the currents in the brain. One version is bulky and uses *superconducting quantum interference devices* which require cooling to −269 °C using liquid helium. Newer experimental versions use an optically *pumped magnetometer* which contains a laser beam and rubidium detectors. The laser beam aligns the rubidium atoms. The magnetic fields in the brain cause perturbations to the atomic alignment resulting in light absorption patterns characteristic of the brain activities which can be detected and analysed. The instrument/scanner is small and uses quantum sensors working at room temperature and the subject wears a helmet containing the sensors.

5.19 Conclusion

The area of neural engineering have been introduced and illustrated by examples from the literature. The useful background material in electromagnetic radiation and wave propagation has been discussed. We note that throughout the book we have been concerned with the *application of electronic engineering in neuroscience and neuromedicine*. The other side of the coin, namely *neuro-inspired electronics*, such as artificial intelligence and neural networks imitating the brain or copying the brain function to design electronic circuits, are not the subject of this book. For a review of these topics from an engineering viewpoint the reader may consult [24], which contains the following articles:

- 'The dawn of the thinking machine'
- 'An engineer's guide to the brain'
- 'The brain as a computer'
- 'What intelligent machines need to learn from the neocortex'
- 'From animal intelligence to artificial intelligence'
- 'Road map for the artificial brain'
- 'The meuromorphic chip's make or break moment'
- 'Navigate like a rat'
- 'Can we quantify machine consciousness?'

References

[1] Akay M (ed) 2001 Special issue on neural engineering: merging engineering and neuroscience *Proc. IEEE* **89** July

[2] Beheshti M and Mottaghy F M (ed) 2003 Special issue on emerging medical imaging technology *Proc. IEEE* **10** November

[3] Ugurbil K *et al* 2001 Magnetic resonance imaging of brain function and neurochemistry *Proc. IEEE* **89** 1093–106 July

[4] Savage N 2008 A weaker cheaper MRI *IEEE Spectr.* **45** 21 January

[5] ChumpusRex 2007 File:Mri scanner schematic labelled.svg *Wikipedia* https://en.wikipedia.org/wiki/File:Mri_scanner_schematic_labelled.svg
[6] Novaksean 2015 File:Normal axial T2-weighted MR image of the brain.jpg *Wikimedia Commons* https://commons.wikimedia.org/wiki/File:Normal_axial_T2-weighted_MR_image_of_the_brain.jpg
[7] Mim.cis 2016 File:T1-weighted-MRI.png *Wikimedia Commons* https://commons.wikimedia.org/wiki/File:T1-weighted-MRI.png
[8] Glazer O 2006 File:Mra1.jpg *Wikimedia Commons* https://commons.wikimedia.org/wiki/File:Mra1.jpg
[9] National Heart Lung and Blood Insitute (NIH) 2013 File:Carotid ultrasound.jpg *Wikimedia Commons* https://commons.wikimedia.org/wiki/File:Carotid_ultrasound.jpg
[10] Drickey 2006 File:ColourDopplerA.jpg *Wikimedia Commons* https://commons.wikimedia.org/wiki/File:ColourDopplerA.jpg
[11] Durand D M and Bikson M 2001 Suppression and control of epileptiform activity by electrical stimulation *Proc. IEEE* **89** 1065–82 July
[12] Boulton C 2021 Bypassing paralysis *IEEE Spectr.* **58** 28–33 February
[13] Cheng C H *et al* 2001 In the blink of a silicon eye *IEEE Circuits Devices Mag.* **17** 20–32 May
[14] BC Family Hearing 2016 File:Cochlear-implant.jpg *Wikimedia Commons* https://commons.wikimedia.org/wiki/File:Cochlear-implant.jpg
[15] Someya T 2013 Building bionic skin *IEEE Spectr.* **50** 44–9 September
[16] Leventon W 2002 Synthetic skin *IEEE Spectr.* **39** 28–33 December
[17] Tyler D J 2016 Restoring the human touch *IEEE Spectr.* **53** 24–9 May
[18] Rosen J and Hannaford B 2006 Doc at a distance *IEEE Spectr.* **43** 28–33 October
[19] Gagnon-Turcotte G *et al* 2020 Smart autonomous electro-optic platforms enabling innovative brain therapies *IEEE Circuits Syst. Mag.* **20** 28–46
[20] Berger T W *et al* 2001 Brain-implantable biomimetic electronics as the next era in neural prosthetics *Proc. IEEE* **89** 993 July
[21] Strickland E 2022 Zapping the brain could treat long Covid *IEEE Spectr.* **59** 9–11 February
[22] Dutta B 2022 Eavesdropping on the brain *IEEE Spectr.* **59** 31–6 June
[23] Choi C Q 2022 A guide to the quantum sensor boom *IEEE Spectr.* **59** 5–7 June
[24] Special Report 2017 Can we copy the brain? *IEEE Spectr.* **54** 21–69 June

www.ingramcontent.com/pod-product-compliance
Ingram Content Group UK Ltd.
Pitfield, Milton Keynes, MK11 3LW, UK
UKHW051848100926
8556IPUK00005B/512

9 780750 334259